Walking the Baby Beat

Answers to Hundreds of Your Healthcare Questions

by
D. Gary Benfield, M.D.

Smart Start Press

To purchase copies of *Walking the Baby Beat* you can do so in any of the following ways:

    Phone: 1-800-247-6553
    Fax: 419-281-6883
    e-Mail: www.atlasbooks.com

Copyright © 2006, D. Gary Benfield, M.D.
                 Smart Start Press

ISBN 0-9779848-0-X
      978-0-9779848-0-0

LCCN 2006902503

The information contained in this book is not intended to substitute for your own doctor's medical advice. Readers should always consult their doctors or other professionals for advice and treatment. The author and the publisher disclaim any liability arising directly or indirectly from the use of this book.

All rights reserved. No part of this book may be reproduced or transmitted in any form or by any means, electronic or mechanical, including photocopying, recording, or by information storage and retrieval systems, without the written permission of the publisher, except by a reviewer who may quote brief passages in a review.

Printed in the United States of America

Table of Contents

Foreword   xiii
Introduction   xvii
Acknowledgments   xxiii

Planning your pregnancy   1
  Is a pre-pregnancy checkup worth the extra effort?   1
  Future mother plans ahead for healthy baby   3
  Folic acid reduces risk of birth defects   4
  Outlook improves for infants of diabetic mothers   5
  Diabetics need counseling before pregnancy   7
  Will lithium affect our baby when my wife becomes pregnant?   8
  What is a genetics counselor?   9
  Will my multiple sclerosis endanger our baby?   9
  Cats in the home and pregnancy may not mix   10
  New hope for lupus and pregnancy   11
  Folic acid–inhibiting drugs increase risk of birth defects   11

Fetal concerns   13
  Is Prozac safe during pregnancy?   13
  Does Accutane cause birth defects?   14
  Can Accutane still cause birth defects after treatment is stopped?   14
  Can an electric shock harm the fetus?   15
  Will Synthroid harm my unborn baby?   16
  Monitoring pregnancy with fetal ultrasound   16
  Is it safe to have sex during pregnancy?   18
  Is it safe to remove a tattoo while pregnant?   18
  Do pregnant smokers put their babies at risk?   19
  Is it safe to drink coffee during pregnancy?   20

Herbal remedies and pregnancy 21
Should pregnant women be tested for HIV? 22

Fetal growth and development 23
Sperm or egg: Which one decides a baby's sex? 24
Gestational age is not the same as conceptual age 24
Intrauterine growth retardation 25
Does the fetus breathe in the womb? 26
Critical periods of fetal development 27

Childbirth 30
Elective C-section or vaginal delivery:
   Which gamble should you take? 30
Some babies take longer to adjust at birth 32
What is a doula? 34
Is labor longer for women who deliver boys? 37
Anticipating problems at birth is good care 37
Emergency childbirth can happen to anyone 38
Signs of birth injury might not show up right away 39
Using a suction cup to complete delivery 40
Writing a birth plan 41
Did my pediatrician charge too much? 43
All you ever wanted to know about cesarean birth 45
Delivery room motto: Be prepared! 47
The cesarean section rate keeps going up 49
Water birth: Dangerous fad or empowering ritual? 52
What happens if my pregnancy goes too long? 54

Storing cord blood 54
Storing cord blood offers peace of mind, at a price 54

Premature baby care 57
If Jackie Kennedy's premature son, Patrick,
   were born today, would he survive? 57
The alphabet soup of premature baby care 59
Facing the challenge of premature birth 61
Massage therapy helps preemies grow 63

"Kangaroo care" helps parents, preemies bond	64
Treating jaundice of prematurity with fluorescent light	65
How do you tell whether a baby is premature or full term?	67

Your newborn by the numbers — 69
- How's your newborn IQ? — 69
- Your newborn by the numbers — 71

Circumcision — 72
- Should we have our baby circumcised? — 72
- How do you take care of the uncircumcised penis? — 74

Twins and higher multiples — 75
- The case of the vanishing twin — 75
- Raising identical twins — 76
- Delivered, but still pregnant — 77
- All twins are not born equal — 78
- Fun facts about celebrity twins — 80

Genetics and birth defects — 83
- Can two brown-eyed parents have a child with blue eyes? — 83
- What happens to the removed fluid after an amniocentesis? — 84
- What are my baby's chances of having Down syndrome? — 85
- Can you explain the fragile X syndrome? — 85
- When cousins plan to marry — 87
- The risk of having a second baby with cystic fibrosis — 88
- What is the life expectancy of children with Down syndrome? — 89
- What are my baby's chances of inheriting sickle cell disease? — 90
- Breaking bad news — 91

Why is my heart on the left side of my chest?	94
Folic acid or folate: Which prevents birth defects best?	96
Not all birth defects show up at birth	99
Why is this two-day-old turning blue with feeding?	100

Breastfeeding your baby   102

Is breastfeeding safe when mom has the flu?	102
Vaccinating your breastfeeding infant	102
Is Amoxicillin safe for breastfeeding mothers?	102
Do breast implants interfere with breastfeeding?	103
The let-down reflex	104
Is propanolol safe for breastfeeding mothers?	105
Should women breastfeed in public?	105
Do breastfed babies grow up smarter?	105
Freezing breast milk for later use is easy	106
Is breastfeeding a reliable contraceptive?	108
Is breastfeeding easier the second time around?	109
Does breastfeeding lower the risk of breast cancer?	110
Is phenobarbital safe for nursing mothers?	110
Do nursing babies have more bowel movements, even later on?	111
Breastfeeding and heavy coffee drinking may not mix	112
Is Prozac safe for nursing mothers?	113

Bleeding concerns in infants   115

The circumcision that won't stop bleeding	115
Vaginal bleeding in the newborn	117
Why is this six-week-old suddenly so sick?	118

Infant air travel   120

Is air travel safe for healthy newborns?	120

Preventing sudden infant death   121
   Important changes in guidelines to prevent SIDS   121
   Babies need tummy time too   124
   Isn't side sleeping for babies a good compromise?   124

Growth and development after birth   125
   Will our 14-month-old ever walk?   125
   Father prays for left-handed son   126
   Eight-month-old has no teeth   127
   Toe-sucking son has parents worried   127
   No crawling for this child   128
   Three-month-old doesn't cry much   128
   Why is this child such a daddy's girl?   129
   When a five-month-old drools and blows bubbles   129
   Will our ten-month-old walk sooner wearing shoes?   130
   When to introduce infants to picture books   130
   How infants feel about strangers   131
   The dad difference in child development   132
   Why won't this seven-month-old eat baby food?   134
   Why do babies sleep differently than adults?   136
   Is this baby's sleeping behavior abnormal?   139
   Giving temperament its due   139
   Coping with colic   140

Parenting   142
   When does love begin?   142
   Helping a child adjust to a new sibling   144
   When a 15-month-old urinates in the bath water   145
   Should fathers share in their babies' care?   147
   "Read me a story"   148
   Babies need parents' attention, not just games and toys   149
   These parents still read aloud to their six-year-old   150
   Choosing your baby's first sitter   151

You are not a bad mother if you bottle feed	152
Helping a choking infant	153
Responding to a baby's cry	154
Why won't this three-month-old stop crying?	156
To work or not to work	157
What parents should know about fever	159
Avoiding "baby bottle tooth decay"	161
Is my baby's tear duct blocked?	161
Does my baby need a daily bath?	162
Do infants need extra vitamins?	163
Most heart murmurs in children are "innocent"	164
What is the appropriate room temperature for a baby?	165
Your baby's soft spot is stronger than you think	165
Taking your baby's temperature	166
Brushing up on healthy teeth	167

Grandparenting — 168

Understanding your new grandchild	168
First-time grandmother	170
Children of lesbian, gay parents	171
Can't doctors and nurses speak English?	172
Grandparents can make a difference	174

Immunizations — 176

Child's cold not a good reason to postpone shots	176
Are all those shots really necessary?	176
Is it important to immunize your child against chicken pox?	177
Routine smallpox vaccination no longer available	179

Toddler time — 180

Our toddler is driving us nuts!	180
When toddlers discover their genitals	181
Tired toddler's self-comforting habit	183
How much TV should a toddler watch?	183
When a toddler has bad breath	185

Is this toddler's heart beating too fast? 186
Toddlers get appendicitis too 186

Infectious diseases 187
What's the difference between a cold and the flu? 187
Overuse of antibiotics can be harmful 190
How does swimmer's ear differ from otitis media? 192
Are pet iguanas safe for children? 195
Chlamydia infection during pregnancy 197
Is there a cure for genital herpes? 197
Do childhood ear infections need antibiotics? 199
Learning from the scars of chickenpox 201
DEET is best for fighting mosquitoes 203
Do cough suppressants work in children
  with a cold? 204

Skin conditions 207
What to do about diaper rash 207
Recognizing and treating cradle cap 209
What are mongolian spots? 209
Are these the bruises of child abuse? 210
Most hemangiomas don't need treatment 212
What's the difference between impetigo and
  ringworm? 212
What causes the rash of poison ivy? 213

Abdominal disorders 214
What is an intussusception? 214
What is necrotizing enterocolitis? 215
Abdominal pain and vomiting: A new twist 217

Child safety 219
A swallowed coin can be dangerous 219
Are infant walkers too dangerous? 220
Do swimming lessons prevent drowning? 221
Does this crib meet modern safety standards? 222
Grim reality of missing and abducted children 224

Preventing abduction: A guide for parents	227
Crawling infants lead dangerous lives	228
Is it safe to burn candles in your bedroom?	230

Day care — 232
What health problems exclude a child from day care? — 232

Child abuse — 233
It's never okay to shake a baby — 233
Shaken baby cases can be difficult to prove — 234
Was this child's injury really accidental? — 236

Cerebral palsy — 238
Do infants outgrow cerebral palsy? — 238
Does hyperbaric oxygen help cerebral palsy? — 238

Sun protection — 240
What does the SPF on sunscreen lotions mean? — 240
Protecting children from the sun — 240
Does an African-American baby need sun protection? — 242
What is adequate sun protection? — 243

Autism — 243
Where can we find reliable information about autism? — 243

Loss of a Child — 244
Remembering our deceased children — 244
Why is the newborn autopsy so important? — 246
Trying again after a newborn death — 248
When a baby dies, forget the free advice — 250
Should a child be allowed to touch her deceased baby brother? — 250

A nurse pulled the curtain between this mother
 and her dying baby 251
Should parents talk about death with their
 dying child? 254

School health 256
Nit-picking about head lice 256

Teen health concerns 260
Children with diabetes can play any sport if . . . 260
When a tubal pregnancy mimics appendicitis 261
Should we let our son go for beach week? 262
Teen health and the law 263
Should teens be included in discussions about
 their health? 264
What is an emancipated minor? 264
Is my 13-year-old's blood pressure normal? 266
Gonorrhea in teens: A sneaky, often silent disease 267
Discussing pregnancy prevention with teens 269
Keys to lifelong bone health 271
Ecstasy is nothing to rave about 273
Does obesity run in families? 274
Childhood obesity and diabetes often go hand
 in hand 276
Is obesity surgery a good idea for teens? 278
When a teenager is genetically different from
 her peers 280
What is meant by heat-related illness? 282
Are 16-year-olds mature enough to drive a car? 285

Ethical issues 287
Should family members be allowed in the
 room during CPR? 287
Would you try to conceive a baby to save a
 sibling's life? 289
Are we doing the right thing? 292

Should the medical team have tried to separate these conjoined twins?	293
When a cure for mother's cancer threatens her unborn baby	294
Should the federal government fund embryonic stem cell research?	297
When a child with Down syndrome outlives his parents	299
Baby's resuscitation raises troubling ethical issues	300

Bonus section
My heroes — 305

The Newborn APGAR Score: Just one of Dr. Virginia Apgar's many achievements	306
Dr. Albert Schweitzer: The renowned humanitarian who showed me the way	314
The hidden talent of Dr. Spock	322
Frieda Pushnik: "The armless and legless wonder"	326
Franklin Delano Roosevelt: Rescued at birth	328
Dr. Ignaz Semmelweis: "You must wash your hands!"	329
Dr. Martin A. Couney: The "incubator-baby doctor"	338
Suddenly paraplegic, Joseph Stock never gave up	343

Resource Center — 345

Index — 357

Foreword

I must admit my bias in writing the "Foreword" to *Walking the Baby Beat*, for I am the author's daughter. So when you hear me say, "This is a great book!" you may naturally think, "Yeah, sure! It's your dad's book!" However, I am also in the lucky position to read this book as a physician and as a mother.

I have counseled my patients as they planned their pregnancies, worried with them as their sons and daughters fought illnesses, all the while dealing with my own insecurities of parenting two young children.

There are parts of this book that I wish every one of my patients could read, parts from which each of my colleagues at work could benefit, and many sections that have already helped guide me and my husband (also a physician) on this roller coaster ride of parenting.

Walking the Baby Beat can be described as a medical resource. It can also be depicted as a "how-to" guide to parenting. History enthusiasts will enjoy the nuggets of trivia sprinkled throughout the book. The concluding section of stories will amaze and inspire. This book will mean different things to different people. As a physician, a mother, and a daughter, here is what it means to me:

As a Family Medicine physician providing obstetrical care, I have the privilege of caring for entire families; from the developing fetus to our great-grandparents. What I cherish most, I think, is when I have the opportunity to help a couple throughout the entire childbearing experience—from planning a pregnancy, to monitoring the prenatal course and delivering the baby, to caring for this baby and family over time. From this medical perspective, *Walking the Baby Beat* is an invaluable resource that addresses the myriad of questions that often arise during these exciting times. Many of the readers' questions are ones I've heard in my examination rooms or even in the doctor's lounge. The information presented is current, understandable, and practical. In this way, this is a rich resource for health care providers and parents alike.

I am also reading this book as the mother of a toddler and an infant. As such, I have wrestled with breastfeeding, endured sleepless nights watching my baby struggle with a cold, questioned whether or not I should continue my job, and battled my toddler over which sippy cup (Cinderella or Nemo) we will use. I have done all of this, like any parent, in the hopes that I can raise two happy and healthy girls. In *Walking the Baby Beat*, we have the comfort of turning to a seasoned physician for explanations of complex medical issues or the comfort of looking to a grandfather for a practical approach to introducing your baby to baby food.

Lastly, and by far most special to me, is that I read this book as the author's daughter. For thirty-two years, I have watched my father walk the baby beat. Granted, it took me a few years to realize that he was not a helicopter pilot, for he told me that, sometimes, he flew in helicopters taking sick babies to the hospital. When I was young, my dad would take my sisters and me to the nursery at the hospital, where we would see rows of incubators housing babies who were learning how to breathe and how to feed.

As I got older, I began to realize that not all babies go to the neonatal intensive care unit before going home. More importantly, I realized that my dad's patients were not only these delicate infants, but also were the families anxiously hovering over their youngest family member, wanting so much to bring him home. Now, as a mother, I watch my father hold my girls, patient and loving, with a knowing and an understanding that only someone who has lived a life around babies could have.

Before reading this book, I thought I had a pretty good understanding of how my dad began on this journey. I knew he read a book by Albert Schweitzer that influenced him to apply to medical school. I had heard that, somewhere along the way, there was a doctor who showed him how to examine newborns in the hospital. I even knew there was a stamp commemorating the achievements of Dr. Virginia Apgar. But I don't think I ever really listened to these stories. In the "My Heroes" section of the book, these stories, along with others, are presented. For me, this section is a wonderful gift. I get to learn about the people and experiences that have helped mold my dad into a father and physician for whom my respect and admiration run so very deep. For you, I hope it will give you a bit of inspiration and that delicious sense of wonder, for these are people who were fortunate enough to find their passion and then live it.

So, for me, this book is, in fact, much more than a parenting guidebook or a medical resource. It is a story, rather many stories, of happiness, tragedy, laughter, and inspiration. It is a story of life!

Cynthia Kelley, D.O.

Introduction

I took my first tentative steps walking the baby beat back in 1964, during the summer between my junior and senior years of medical school. That's when Dr. Bob Irwin, a Baltimore pediatrician, invited me up to the nursery at the old South Baltimore General Hospital. Then he did something I'll never forget: he rolled up his sleeves, scrubbed his hands, and showed me how to examine a brand new baby, complete with running commentary.

He said. "This is the most important physical this baby will ever have. Always keep that in mind."

He said, "Be gentle, and talk to the baby as you go along. You'll be amazed how a baby will turn to your voice and follow you with her eyes."

He said, "Be systematic and thorough. Start from the head and work down, or start from the feet and work up. But do it the same way every time."

He said, "You haven't done a complete exam until you've run your fingers over every square inch of the baby's body. That way, you won't miss anything."

He said, "Be sure to count the baby's fingers and toes. There's nothing more embarrassing than having a mother tell you, the doctor, that her baby is missing a toe or has an extra finger."

He said, "Don't try to force a baby's eyes open with your fingers. Pick her up under her arms and glide her slowly from side to side. Her eyes will open automatically. Then you can get a good look."

He said, "If you hear what you think are strange breath sounds, remove your stethoscope from the baby's chest and listen in front of her nose. If you hear the same sounds, chances are you were only hearing transmitted nasal sounds."

He said, "Try to do each baby's first exam in the mother's room. She can see what you're doing and ask questions as you go along."

He said, "When you've finished examining the baby, don't stand and talk down to the baby's mother. Pull up a chair and have a face-to-face conversation."

When Dr. Irwin was finished, we switched places. Then he patiently talked me through my very first newborn physical exam.

Of course, I was clumsy. Of course, the baby peed on my gown. And, of course, I had to change his diaper when I was done. But I was so elated, none of that mattered.

You might say I was hooked!

After graduating from medical school, I completed three years of residency training in pediatrics and served two years in the U.S. Air Force as a pediatrician. Then I focused on newborns, taking a two-year fellowship in the brand new specialty of neonatology—newborn intensive care—at Cincinnati Children's Hospital. I arrived at Akron Children's Hospital in August 1972, where I've walked the baby beat ever since.

In 1972, most babies born with a surgically repairable birth defect were a surprise in the delivery room. That's because obstetricians and family doctors lacked the tools they have today to diagnose the birth defect early in pregnancy and anticipate problems at birth.

So it was not uncommon to get called out in the middle of the night to help stabilize a distressed baby and to figure out why the baby was having difficulty. A whole team of specialists–pediatric surgeon, radiologist, neonatologist, and others–would put our heads together like good baby detectives and try to figure out the diagnosis. Then the surgeon would whisk the baby off to the operating room.

Today, things are different. Most major birth defects are diagnosed before birth, thanks to advances in technology such as fetal ultrasound, amniocentesis, and fetal echocardiography, which allows the cardiologist to see the baby's beating heart and diagnose most heart problems well before the baby is born.

One of the fascinating things about the baby beat is you never know what's coming next. For instance:

- I've taken care of seriously ill newborns and their anxious parents in the Neonatal Intensive Care Unit at Akron Children's Hospital, where we've ridden that emotional roller coaster together many times.
- I've lain awake at night, especially after a baby has died, and wondered over and over if some other doctor, somewhere else, might have been able to do a better job, perhaps saving that baby's life.
- I've taken care of healthy babies and their mothers in the well baby nurseries at the adult hospitals in Akron. Oftentimes, our biggest challenge was deciding whether or not to circumcise the baby or how to get mom's breast milk flowing.
- I've taken care of babies born to teenage moms who've dropped out of school and seemed lost. Their goal in life seemed to focus in on just having fun. "My mom will take care of the baby, if he lives."
- On the other hand, I've also taken care of babies born to teenage moms who have stayed in school. I would find them at their baby's bedside, catching up on their missed assignments in math, physics, history, or English. And with their parents' help, they planned on raising their babies and going on to college.
- I've also met with anxious parents after they've learned their unborn baby was afflicted with a serious birth defect and would need surgery shortly after birth. Part of my task was to help them understand what to expect after their baby was born, to help them make decisions about their baby's care, and to plan for the baby's birth.

I've also been in the delivery room when all three of our daughters were born. And, yes, I've counted their fingers and toes and listened to their chests. And when I heard the lub-dub, lub-dub, lub-dub of their beating hearts, it sounded to me like God's voice speaking.

I've helped raise our daughters through childhood, adolescence, and college. (They do grow up, don't they?) And I've walked all three of them down the aisle, wondering each time if the young man we were walking toward was good enough for the special woman on my arm.

I've held three granddaughters within minutes after their births. I've savored those moments, each time grateful that all went well.

Nine years ago, my walk took another turn when I started writing a weekly newspaper column, The Baby Beat, for *The Alliance Review*. In the column, I answer questions from readers on a wide variety of topics, (not just about babies) ranging from planning your pregnancy to childbirth to teen health concerns. Most of the material for *Walking The Baby Beat* has been drawn from those updated columns.

Walking The Baby Beat is easy to use. Each topic is arranged chronologically, starting with "Planning Your Pregnancy" and ending with "Teen Health Concerns." In addition, the title of each specific problem or question is listed in the extensive table of contents. Simply check the table of contents or consult the index to find the specific problems or questions that interest you most. Or, once you get started, who knows, perhaps you may want to read the book straight through.

As an added bonus, *Walking The Baby Beat* introduces you to eight outstanding people, five of them medical pioneers, in a special section called "My Heroes."

When I encountered this cast of colorful and intriguing characters, I discovered I had more in common with them than I ever thought possible. Then, when I realized their journeys were much like my own, I had this incredible "Aha!" That discovery helped change my life.

Perhaps, when you read their stories, you'll have a similar "Aha!"

So, welcome to *Walking The Baby Beat*. I'm so glad to have you along.

A further thought: In February 2001, I was thumbing through the latest issue of the *American Academy of Pediatrics News* when I came across a picture of Bob Irwin. His hair was gray and balding in front, but his smile hadn't changed. The caption read: "Robert C. Irwin, M.D. of Baltimore, died of a heart attack Nov. 1, 2000, at age 68."

As I stared at the picture, I had one regret: If only I had thanked him one more time before he was gone.

So now I'll say it: Thank you, Bob, for introducing me to the wonderful world of newborns and for starting me off in the right direction. I'll always remember your special gift.

D. Gary Benfield, M.D.

Acknowledgments

I have dedicated this book to my parents, Robert and Minnie Benfield, who gave my brother, Eric, and me their unconditional love and support for as long as they lived. All they ever asked of us was to do our best.

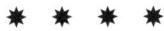

I would also like to thank the following:

- G. Charles Dix II, publisher of *The Alliance Review*, for giving me the opportunity, nine years ago, to write The Baby Beat, my own weekly newspaper column.
- James R. Bennett of Homestead Publishing Company, for introducing me to the world of book publishing and urging me to write this book.
- My wife, Cathy, for thoughtfully taking her red pen to my draft columns, week after week, for the past nine years.
- Ted Stevens, medical photographer in the Audio-Visual Department at Akron Children's Hospital, for taking the photographs appearing on the front and back cover of this book.
- My granddaughters, Sarah Noelle Kelley and Emma Grace Kelley, who appear in those same photos.
- My medical and nursing colleagues in Akron, for teaching me so much while walking the baby beat together.
- The thousands of parents I've encountered while walking the baby beat, for sharing your inspiring stories and showing me what it's like to walk in your shoes.

Planning your Pregnancy

IS A PRE-PREGNANCY CHECKUP WORTH THE EXTRA EFFORT?

Q *My husband and I have been married for three years and are ready to start our family. I want to make an appointment with an obstetrician to talk about it first. My husband thinks it's too much trouble and just wants to see whether I can get pregnant. Can you explain to me so I can explain to him why it might be important to meet with the doctor first?*

A It's astonishing that so many couples would attempt to get pregnant and have a baby without any planning whatsoever. "If my wife gets pregnant, fine. But if she doesn't, we'll try again next month." Or, worse yet: "You're pregnant? Now what are we going to do?"

So, thank you for the opportunity to discuss pre-pregnancy planning, not just because 50 percent of all pregnancies in this country are unplanned, but because pre-pregnancy planning can really matter to your future baby's health.

If you and your spouse decide the time is right to try to get pregnant, you should schedule a pre-pregnancy appointment for the two of you to meet with your obstetrician.

One of the things the doctor will ask you both is about your family medical histories. You can save a lot of time and have more accurate information if you put together a medical family tree before your appointment.

Some health conditions, such as diabetes, high blood pressure, and seizure disorders tend to run in families. If a close relative, especially a sibling, a parent, or a grandparent has a certain condition, you or your baby could be at greater risk of having it.

Certain medical conditions are genetic disorders, meaning they're passed from parent to child through DNA.

D. Gary Benfield, M.D.

Examples include sickle cell anemia, cystic fibrosis, and muscular dystrophy. Even if you don't have the disorder itself, you may carry the mutation in your genes and pass it along to your baby.

Typically, your pre-pregnancy appointment will also include a thorough physical exam. You may also have blood tests to check your immunity to certain infections such as chickenpox (varicella) and German measles (rubella). If you aren't immune, your doctor will probably vaccinate you, because both diseases can cause serious birth defects or illness in your baby.

If you have an ongoing health condition such as diabetes, asthma, or high blood pressure, it's best to have it under control before you get pregnant. This precaution reduces the risks for both you and your baby.

You may also be taking medication for a health condition, such as phenobarbital or Dilantin for a seizure disorder; Prozac or Paxil for depression; or Accutane for cystic acne. Accutane should never be prescribed for women who are or may become pregnant. The risk to the baby of causing a severe birth defect clearly outweighs any benefit. In fact, the manufacturer requires a negative serum pregnancy test two weeks before beginning therapy.

Your doctor will also ask about previous pregnancies. This information is especially important if a previous pregnancy was complicated by high blood pressure, diabetes, the birth of a premature baby, or a baby born with a birth defect.

Your doctor will also remind you that no amount of smoking or alcohol consumption has been proven safe during pregnancy.

The doctor will also suggest that you start taking a multivitamin that contains 0.4 milligrams of folic acid before you get pregnant. If you wait until your pregnancy test turns positive to start taking folic acid, it may be too late to reduce the risk of a neural tube defect, such as spina bifida.

Well, these are just some of the potential benefits of pre-pregnancy planning. What do you think? Is it worth the extra effort for your future baby's sake?

I think so.

FUTURE MOTHER PLANS AHEAD FOR HEALTHY BABY

Q *I'm 26 and engaged to a wonderful guy. We've planned our wedding for a year from now. The only problem is I'm almost 60 pounds over my ideal weight. I'm working hard to lose as much as I can before the wedding, but not because I don't like the way I look. It's mainly because we plan on starting our family soon after we get married and want to have a healthy baby. Does that plan make sense to you?*

A It makes perfect sense to me for several reasons. First, you've obviously done your homework. Compared to women of normal weight, women who are obese at the time of conception have twice the risk of giving birth to babies with heart defects and three times the risk of delivering babies with open spine defects or the abdominal malformation known as omphalocele, in which the intestines and other abdominal organs protrude into the umbilical cord, according to the Centers for Disease Control and Prevention (CDC).

Moreover, pre-pregnancy obesity is a major cause of premature births in the United States, according to the March of Dimes.

A recent study from Denmark shows that pre-pregnancy obesity is associated with an increased risk of stillbirth, especially late in pregnancy. So yes, by losing weight, you are doing all you can to have a healthy baby.

But, there's more to it than that. You're also looking out for your own health by lowering your risk for heart disease, stroke, sleep apnea, type II diabetes, gallbladder disease, certain types of cancer, depression, and arthritis, all associated with obesity. Lastly, you are doing something even lovebirds Tom Cruise and Katie Holmes couldn't do, waiting until after marriage to start your family.

Congratulations!

FOLIC ACID REDUCES RISK OF BIRTH DEFECTS

Q *My wife's best friend recently gave birth to a baby with an open spine defect. Now, my wife is worried she might become pregnant and have a baby with the same problem. Can you tell us how open spine defects occur? Can we do anything to prevent them?*

A Yes, your wife and all women of childbearing age can do something to lower the risk of "open spine" defects. But first, let me explain how these defects occur.

Early in pregnancy, near the 20th day after conception, a tiny groove, called the neural groove, forms on the backside of the developing embryo. At this point, the embryo is only about two to three millimeters long. (If you have a Roosevelt dime handy, this length is the same as Roosevelt's nose.)

Normally, the neural groove closes on the 28th day after conception and becomes the neural tube—the forerunner of our spinal column and brain. (If you trace a line from the tip of your tail bone up the middle of your back and neck and continue forward to the center of your forehead, this imaginary line marks your closed neural tube.)

In one out of 1,000 pregnancies, the neural tube fails to close completely, resulting in a neural tube defect, or NTD.

When the neural tube fails to close at the embryo's tail end, the result is spina bifida or an "open spine" defect. Most likely, this type of defect was the one that affected your wife's friend's child. Shortly after birth, these babies require surgery to close their open spine.

Babies born with an open spine may also develop hydrocephalus, commonly known as water on the brain, and need a second operation to drain the extra fluid. Later on, these children have serious disabilities. Their legs and feet are often paralyzed, and they have problems with bowel and bladder control.

When the neural tube fails to close at the embryo's head end, the skull fails to close and the incompletely formed brain shows through. Babies born with this condition, known as anencephaly, all die before or shortly after birth.

Each year in the United States, approximately 4,000 pregnancies are affected by NTDs, and more than 2,500 babies are born with this problem. NTDs cause more than 500 infant deaths annually, not counting the 1,500 or so babies who are aborted after the diagnosis is made by ultrasound.

The good news is that 50 to 70 percent of all NTDs can be prevented if all women of childbearing age regularly take a multivitamin tablet that contains 0.4 mg of folic acid. Because more than half of all pregnancies in the United States are unplanned and neural tube defects occur early in pregnancy, it's crucial to start taking a multivitamin supplement before becoming pregnant.

A further thought: Folate, the naturally occurring form of folic acid, is found in green leafy vegetables, beans, asparagus, citrus fruits, whole grain foods, and liver. However, it's difficult to get enough folate through diet alone. You can make up the difference and get maximum protection against neural tube defects by taking a multivitamin supplement daily.

OUTLOOK IMPROVES FOR INFANTS OF DIABETIC MOTHERS

Q *My husband and I have been married almost five years, and now we want to start a family. But here's the hitch: I have taken insulin for diabetes for the past 16 years, since I* *was 12. Can we anything do to improve our chances of having a healthy baby?*

A Now, before you become pregnant, is the best time to ask. Here's why.

Years ago, the death toll for infants of diabetic mothers was remarkably high. The reasons? A large number of stillbirths late in pregnancy and a large number of babies born with birth defects.

In response to the large number of late-pregnancy stillbirths, obstetricians started delivering infants of diabetic mothers early, and it worked. But the trade-off was more premature births and complications of prematurity.

Then, researchers discovered that if diabetic women strictly controlled their blood sugars while pregnant, they could not only lower the risk of stillbirth, but they could carry their pregnancies closer to term.

More recently, researchers discovered a new approach: If insulin-dependent diabetic women get their blood sugar levels under strict control before becoming pregnant, not only can they reduce the number of late-pregnancy stillbirths and carry their pregnancies closer to term, they can also lower the risk of birth defects to that of nondiabetic women.

This "preconception" approach to managing diabetes improves the chances of having healthier babies and all but replaces the need for repeated hospitalizations during pregnancy to regulate maternal blood sugar.

So you see, there's a lot you can do to increase your chances of having a healthy baby. It all begins by asking your doctor for more details before becoming pregnant.

A further thought: Before Drs. Banting and Best discovered insulin in 1922, 50 percent of pregnant diabetics died during their pregnancies, and the outlook for their babies was even gloomier. Of the babies who escaped death early in pregnancy from miscarriage or premature birth, 50 percent were either stillborn or died from birth defects in the newborn period. Today, thanks to medical progress, women living with diabetes have much more to look forward to than their sisters did 75 years ago, before the discovery of insulin.

DIABETICS NEED COUNSELING BEFORE PREGNANCY

Q *I am 26, have a great job, and am married to a wonderful man. We want to start a family. But I have taken insulin for diabetes for years. I recently read an ad claiming that fenugreek, an herb grown in southern Europe, is good for diabetes and could possibly eliminate my need to take insulin. If true, that would be a godsend. Before I try it, can you tell me whether fenugreek is safe to take during pregnancy?*

A Hold on, let's take first things first. Until a few years ago, diabetics who became pregnant had an increased risk of having problems with their pregnancies. But all of that changed with the advent of counseling prior to conception.

Studies show that when insulin-dependent diabetics sit down with their obstetrician before they get pregnant and plan their pregnancy, their risk of having a problem pregnancy (including problems for the baby) is no greater than that of women who don't have diabetes. Now, that's a godsend!

Preconceptual counseling involves optimizing your diet and insulin dose, starting on a multiple vitamin that contains folic acid, doing some blood tests, and arranging for prenatal care once you become pregnant.

You can also use this visit to ask your doctor questions, including the one about fenugreek. The *Botanical Safety Handbook* lists fenugreek as one of those herbs that should not be used during pregnancy (*American Herbal Products*

D. Gary Benfield, M.D.

Association's Botanical Safety Handbook. Edited by Michael McGuffin, 1997 by CRC Press LLC, Boca Raton, FL).

A further thought: The Food and Drug Administration now advises against using St. John's wort if you are also taking one of many drugs used to treat the following:

- Heart disease (drugs such as digoxin, diltiazem, nifedipine, digitoxin, or beta blockers)
- Depression (drugs such as imipramine, amoxapine, or amitriptyline)
- Seizures (drugs such as carbamazepine, Dilantin, or phenobarbital)
- Cancer (drugs such as cyclophosphamide, tamoxifen, Taxol, or etoposide)

It seems St. John's wort causes these drugs to be eliminated too quickly from the body, making them less effective. Likewise, St. John's wort has the same effect on birth control pills, making them less effective and increasing the chances for an unwanted pregnancy.

WILL LITHIUM AFFECT OUR BABY WHEN MY WIFE BECOMES PREGNANT?

Q *My wife takes lithium for a manic-depressive disorder. Will the drug affect the baby when she becomes pregnant?*

A Lithium does cause birth defects, mainly involving the heart, in infants born to mothers taking the drug during the first four months of pregnancy. The FDA states that lithium may be used during pregnancy only if, in the opinion of the physician, the potential benefits outweigh the possible risks. Use of the drug near the time of birth may result in a depressed baby, which is usually reversible. In addition, the long-term effects of lithium exposure on the baby have not been studied.

The two of you should make an appointment with your wife's doctor for preconceptual counseling.

A further thought: Lithium is excreted into breast milk. The American Academy of Pediatrics recommends that breast-feeding mothers not take lithium because of the potential for lithium-induced toxicity in the nursing infant. This issue should also be discussed when you sit down with your doctor for preconceptual counseling.

WHAT IS A GENETICS COUNSELOR?

Q *My husband and I are ready to start having children, but both sides of our family have a history of birth defects. My doctor suggests we see a genetics counselor. Can you tell me what a genetics counselor does and where we can find one?*

A Genetics counselors are trained to take family histories, gather information from hospital records, and then present families with genetic facts and choices in a neutral manner. They usually work as part of a team under the direction of an M.D. or Ph.D. geneticist.

Most medical schools and some large hospitals now have departments of medical genetics or are associated with a university genetics department. You can write to the March of Dimes, 1275 Mamaroneck Avenue, White Plains, New York, 10605, or visit the March of Dimes Web site (www.marchofdimes.com) for the address and telephone number of the nearest genetics center.

WILL MY MULTIPLE SCLEROSIS ENDANGER OUR BABY?

Q *Five years ago when I was 25, newly married, and in graduate school, I was diagnosed with multiple sclerosis. At the time, I put my dreams on hold; I needed time to adjust. Now* that I've worked through my grief and accept my disease, I want to start a family. Can you tell me whether my having multiple sclerosis will endanger the baby?

A Research has shown that multiple sclerosis (MS) and pregnancy can coexist without unusual complications for mother or for baby. It's also safe for women with MS to breastfeed their babies. However, because each case of MS is different, it's important that you seek preconceptual counseling with your doctor for further advice.

CATS IN THE HOME AND PREGNANCY MAY NOT MIX

Q *I am trying to get pregnant and just returned from a checkup. I told the nurse that we have two cats, and I take care of them. She kind of winced and said we would probably have to get rid of the cats. Can you explain what having two cats has to do with me being pregnant?*

A Apparently, the nurse forgot to tell you that the parasite that causes toxoplasmosis is excreted in cat feces. (This parasite is also found in undercooked meat.) When you clean the cats' litter box, you may come into contact with this parasite, develop a mild case of toxoplasmosis, and not even know it.

Then, if you become pregnant while the organism is floating around in your system, chances are it will cross the placenta and invade the fetal blood stream and disrupt its developing organs. This parasite thrives on growing brain tissue, including the eyes.

To prevent this, you should ask your husband to take over the chore of cleaning the cats' litter box before you become pregnant and to continue doing it until after the baby is born.

Meanwhile, you should carefully wash your hands each time you handle the cats. If, for some reason, this approach isn't feasible, only then will you have to consider getting rid of the cats.

NEW HOPE FOR LUPUS AND PREGNANCY

Q *My husband and I just celebrated our sixth wedding anniversary. We put off having children until we finished college and got started in our careers. Unfortunately, now that we are ready, I have been recently diagnosed with lupus. Can you tell me whether this mysterious disease will affect our chances of having a healthy baby?*

A Years ago, most medical texts said that lupus patients could not have children, and if they became pregnant, they should have a therapeutic abortion. Nowadays, approximately 50 percent of all lupus pregnancies are completely normal, and 25 percent deliver normal babies prematurely. Fetal loss or death of the baby accounts for the remaining 25 percent. So even though pregnancy with lupus still has its problems, pregnancies are possible, and normal children are the rule.

Before attempting to get pregnant, you should make an appointment with your doctor for preconceptual counseling. Meanwhile, you can call the Lupus Foundation of America at 800-558-0121 to request information about lupus and pregnancy, or go to their Web site at www.lupus.org for a wealth of information.

FOLIC ACID–INHIBITING DRUGS INCREASE THE RISK OF BIRTH DEFECTS

By now, most of us know that women who are regularly taking a multivitamin containing folic acid when they become pregnant lower their risk by two-thirds of having a baby with a neural tube defect.

D. Gary Benfield, M.D.

A study published in the prestigious *New England Journal of Medicine*, however, claims drugs that interfere with the body's use of folic acid increase the risk of a variety of birth defects, not only those that involve the neural tube.

Most drugs that interfere with the body's use of folic acid are known as dihydrofolate reductase inhibitors. They include the following:

- Aminopterin and methotrexate, two cancer drugs
- Sulfasalazine, an anti-inflammatory drug
- Pyrimethamine, used to treat protozoal infections
- Triamterene, a diuretic
- Trimethoprim, an ingredient of the antibiotic Bactrim

Some drugs used to treat epilepsy and a few psychological conditions, including Dilantin, phenobarbital, primidone, and carbamazepine, can also affect folic acid.

Researchers in the study found the following:

- The risk of heart defects tripled, and oral defects such as cleft lip or palate doubled if women used dihydrofolate reductase inhibitors during the first three months of pregnancy.
- The risk of heart, oral, and urinary tract defects doubled if women used the epilepsy medicines.
- However, if women in the study were taking multivitamins that contain folic acid, they reduced most of the extra risk of birth defects among women using the dihydrofolate reductase inhibitors, but not among those taking the epilepsy medicines.
- This difference probably results because the drugs used to treat epilepsy may also have a direct toxic effect on the developing fetus that extra folic acid won't prevent.

So what should women taking one of these drugs do if they want to become pregnant?

Because half of all pregnancies in this country are unplanned (meaning by the time a women discovers she is pregnant, it may be too late to start taking folic acid), the best way to lower the risk of having a baby with one or more of these defects is for women of childbearing age to do two things:

- Regularly take a multivitamin containing folic acid.
- Seek their doctors' advice.

Together, doctor and patient can weigh the risks and benefits to the mother and to the baby of continuing the medication versus stopping or changing it.

It's also important for doctors who prescribe these drugs for a woman of childbearing age to inquire whether she is pregnant and to warn her of the possible consequences should she become pregnant.

Fetal concerns

IS PROZAC SAFE DURING PREGNANCY?

Q *My husband and I have been married for four years, and we would like to start our family. For the past year, I've been taking Prozac for depression. Can Prozac harm the baby? Is it safe to take when breastfeeding?*

A One large study, published in the highly respected *New England Journal of Medicine,* compared pregnant women taking Prozac to pregnant women not taking the drug. The researchers found no difference between the two groups for the number of miscarriages, stillbirths, and babies born with a major birth defect.

However, at least one animal study showed that Prozac can produce changes in the fetal brain. Therefore, the maternal benefits should be carefully weighed against the potential fetal risks before exposing the fetus to this drug.

The issue of breastfeeding while taking Prozac is different. A small amount of Prozac may pass into breast milk, but its safety for breastfeeding babies hasn't been adequately studied.

You and your husband should make an appointment with your doctor for preconceptual counseling.

DOES ACCUTANE CAUSE BIRTH DEFECTS?

Q *My doctor recently prescribed Accutane for my acne, and it really helps. She also warned me it could harm the baby if I got pregnant. I'm concerned because a girlfriend of mine who also takes Accutane says it's safe to use during pregnancy. Can you tell me who is right?*

A Your doctor is correct. Your girlfriend is flirting with danger if she becomes pregnant while taking this useful, but potentially dangerous, drug. Accutane is classified Category X, which means the risk of taking the drug during or immediately before pregnancy clearly outweighs any benefit. The manufacturer of Accutane recommends that women stop using the drug at least one month before trying to become pregnant. Check back with your doctor if you still have concerns.

CAN ACCUTANE STILL CAUSE BIRTH DEFECTS AFTER TREATMENT IS STOPPED?

Q *I'm 20 years old and about to begin my second course of Accutane for treatment of severe acne. I'm aware it can cause birth defects and am taking precautions to avoid such a* calamity. I plan to be married in June, and my fiancé and I very much want a family someday. Can you please tell me whether Accutane can cause birth defects years later after stopping treatment?

A The manufacturer of Accutane, Hoffman-LaRoche, recommends that women taking the drug continue using contraception for one month after stopping therapy. By then, all of the drug should be completely eliminated from a woman's system. After that, the risk of having a baby with a birth defect in a future pregnancy is no greater than that for a woman who never took the drug.

CAN AN ELECTRIC SHOCK HARM THE FETUS?

Q *My pregnant sister recently suffered an electric shock when she touched a faulty toaster. Though she shrugged it off, I'm concerned. If a pregnant woman is accidentally shocked, can it harm the fetus?*

A I found four published reports that described 14 pregnant women who were shocked with alternating current, either 110 volts or 220 volts, from appliances or faulty wiring in the home. In each of the cases, the electric current took a hand-to-foot pattern through the body. Although none of the mothers was injured or even lost consciousness, fetal death occurred in 10. In at least half the cases, fetal movement stopped immediately.

Though the specific cause of fetal death has not been determined, in most instances it was probably due to changes in fetal heart conduction resulting in cardiac arrest. Based on these reports, pregnant women who have suffered an electrical shock should seek immediate medical attention to closely monitor the fetus.

WILL SYNTHROID HARM MY UNBORN BABY?

Q *I take Synthroid for hypothyroidism and just found out I'm pregnant. Can you tell me if my taking Synthroid will adversely affect my baby?*

A On the contrary, because untreated hypothyroid women have an increased risk of stillbirths and miscarriages, you need the Synthroid to maintain normal thyroid function which, in turn, protects your baby. Just be sure your obstetrician is aware of your condition and how much Synthroid you are taking.

MONITORING PREGNANCY WITH FETAL ULTRASOUND

Q *I'm supposed to have my first ultrasound in two weeks. Can you explain how fetal ultrasound works? Is it safe for the baby?*

A To understand how fetal ultrasound works, it helps to know a bit about sound itself. So bear with me for just a moment.

When I strike middle C on the piano, the felt hammer connected to the key strikes a steel wire string, causing the string to vibrate 256 times or cycles per second. The vibrating string creates waves of sound that travel through the surrounding air, also at a frequency of 256 cycles per second. (The frequency of a sound is the number of sound waves that pass a given point each second.)

When the sound waves strike my ear drum, a message is sent to my brain that says, "This sound is middle C." If I strike the key an octave above middle C, that steel wire string vibrates 512 times per second, producing a sound wave double the frequency of middle C.

Walking the Baby Beat

The human ear is capable of hearing sounds with frequencies between 20 and 20,000 cycles per second. Sounds below this range are called subsonic; sounds above this range are called ultrasonic. Thus, ultrasound has a frequency greater than 20,000 cycles per second, beyond the range of human hearing.

Now, back to your question: When doing a fetal ultrasound, the technician applies a palm-sized transducer, which generates pulses of sound between 2 million and 10 million cycles per second, to the pregnant woman's lower abdomen, above her uterus.

The painless pulses of sound penetrate the abdomen, strike the target area—in this case, the fetus within the uterus—and are reflected back to the transducer. The transducer sends the reflected echoes to a computer within the ultrasound machine.

The computer transforms the echoes into visual images of the fetus and surrounding tissues. They then appear on the computer screen. As far as I know, no safety concerns regarding the procedure have been reported.

An ultrasound is often done within the first 12 weeks of pregnancy. This early scanning helps to answer these three questions:

- Is my baby alive?
- How far along is my baby?
- How many babies am I carrying?

Viability is confirmed when the pulsating heart is seen. The earliest age at which the pulsating heart can be seen is five weeks after conception, when the embryo is little more than an eighth-of-an-inch long. Amazing, isn't it?

To scan for gestational age, the technician moves the transducer around to obtain the longest image of the fetus. Then the technician freezes the frame and measures fetal length from end to end.

Most ultrasound machines are programmed to convert this measurement into a gestational age. The technician then compares this measured gestational age with the predicted gestational age based on when mom started her last menstrual period. If the two methods agree within several days, an approximate due date is calculated and given to mom.

Fetal number is determined by scanning the entire uterine cavity from top to bottom and side to side. This step is important so as not to overlook more than one fetus.

A further thought: Don't forget to ask the technician for two copies of the best view of your baby's ultrasound. You can mount one copy in an acrylic frame for display, and place the other on the first page of your baby book.

IS IT SAFE TO HAVE SEX DURING PREGNANCY?

Q *After four years of trying, I am finally pregnant. The problem is I sometimes feel contractions after my husband and I have sex. Can these contractions lead to early labor? Should we stop having sex until after the baby is born? Any insight would be helpful.*

A Normally, it's safe to have sex during pregnancy. It's normal to sometimes notice mild contractions after intercourse. No one knows for sure whether these contractions are caused by breast stimulation, female orgasm, or hormones in the male sperm. You should ask your doctor for guidance.

IS IT SAFE TO REMOVE A TATTOO WHILE PREGNANT?

Q *When I was 17, I got a tattoo on my shoulder. Now I want to have it removed. The problem is I'm 14 weeks pregnant,* *and the dermatologist won't remove it until after the baby is born. Can you tell me why I have to wait?*

A Because many tattoos are removed using a laser, and it's not clear how safe it might be for your baby to have this done during pregnancy. This is probably why your doctor wants you to wait. Makes sense to me.

DO PREGNANT SMOKERS PUT THEIR BABIES AT RISK?

Q *I've been married for 12 years and am happy to say I just learned I am pregnant. The problem is I smoke about a pack of cigarettes a day. Can you tell me how smoking might affect the baby? Maybe it will help me quit.*

A Congratulations on your pregnancy! It must be a marvelous feeling. That feeling alone has motivated thousands upon thousands of women to stop smoking.

Many studies show that cigarette smoking is associated with low birthweight, but the story about how it happens is still incomplete. Why? Because cigarette smoke contains more than 3,000 different chemicals, and we still don't know how each of them affects the growing fetus. Most studies, however, focus on three key ingredients of tobacco smoke:

- Nicotine
- Carbon monoxide
- Cyanide

Nicotine is a powerful vasoconstrictor, meaning it restricts blood flow to the uterus. Reduced blood flow to the uterus means fewer nutrients and less oxygen cross the placenta to reach the baby. The result is stunted fetal growth.

Both carbon monoxide and cyanide can damage cells and directly reduce fetal growth. Carbon monoxide also reduces the amount of oxygen carried by red blood cells.

Women who smoke also tend to consume fewer calories and gain less weight. This lower weight gain contributes to reduced birthweight for the baby.

Smoking during pregnancy is associated with the following adverse effects:

- Higher rates of spontaneous miscarriage
- Premature labor
- Sudden infant death syndrome
- More childhood illnesses and school problems, as well as lower IQ

The good news is that women who quit smoking by the twentieth week of pregnancy usually have babies of similar size and health as women who never smoked.

A further thought: A pregnant woman who smokes should not hide this important fact from her doctor. And, by all means, don't try the nicotine patch without discussing it first with your doctor. In several small studies, nicotine replacement therapy, while not associated with adverse outcomes, did have a short-term effect on fetal breathing movements and fetal heart rate. Your doctor can advise you about the risks and benefits of trying the patch, as well as other ways to help you stop smoking.

IS IT SAFE TO DRINK COFFEE DURING PREGNANCY?

Q *I am three months pregnant and drink three or four cups of regular coffee daily. Can that much caffeine harm the baby? I also plan to breastfeed—does caffeine get into breast milk? If so, can it harm my baby?*

A Like most drugs, caffeine crosses the placenta, enters the fetal blood stream and reaches a level similar to that of the mother. To my knowledge, there are no reports that describe the harmful effects of caffeine on the fetus.

Caffeine is excreted in breast milk, reaching a peak level about an hour after consumption. Irritability and poor sleeping patterns have been observed in nursing infants whose mothers consumed more than twice as much as you do.

The American Academy of Pediatrics says drinking a reasonable amount of caffeinated beverages is compatible with breastfeeding. After your baby is born, you might try spacing out your coffee intake to no more than one cup after every other feeding.

HERBAL REMEDIES AND PREGNANCY

Q *My wife, who is several weeks pregnant, and I both love the tangy mint taste of pennyroyal tea so much that we drink it daily. She also uses pennyroyal oil on her skin. Can you tell us whether pennyroyal is safe for the baby?*

A As you know, the leafy form of pennyroyal can be immersed in hot water to make a tea or the essential oil can be used in a bath, a humidifier or vaporizer, or applied directly to the skin as a source of healing and energy. However, you may not know that pennyroyal has a stimulating effect on the uterus and thus could accidentally cause a miscarriage.

Pennyroyal, in any form, should not be used during pregnancy, according to the American Herbal Products Association. Also, mothers should not use the oil after birth to massage the baby and should be sure to rub off any oil they may have on before breastfeeding. This oil is too strong for a newborn and might easily be transferred from the baby's fingers to the eyes or mouth.

Pennyroyal is one of many herbs to avoid because it may accidentally cause a miscarriage. Here's a list of some others that also fit this category:

- Sage
- Tansy
- Wormwood
- Southernwood
- Thuja
- Black and blue cohash
- Goldenseal

A further thought: Sales of herbal medicines in this country are booming, totaling more than $3 billion annually. Even though millions of Americans are now using herbal medicines, more than half of them don't tell their doctors. And because some doctors are inadequately informed about herbs, they usually don't ask. What then should a woman who uses herbs do if she is contemplating pregnancy or finds herself pregnant?

To be on the safe side, women should not use herbs during the first trimester when the fetus is developing and is most susceptible to anything that might cause birth defects. Women should only use herbs during the rest of their pregnancy after consulting an herbal medicine expert or their healthcare provider.

SHOULD PREGNANT WOMEN BE TESTED FOR HIV?

Q *I'm 32, single, and just found out I'm pregnant. I'm also self-sufficient financially and don't plan on getting married, at least not to the baby's father. My question is this: Should I get an AIDS test when I go for my first prenatal checkup?*

A Yes you should—for your own health, that of your baby, and for the health of your sexual partners. You don't want to become part of an alarming statistic: Of the 900,000 Americans living with HIV today, one out of four do not know they are infected.

This lack of knowledge means that these people are not getting the antiretroviral medication that can improve and prolong their lives, and that they are unwittingly capable of infecting their sexual partners. When an infected woman becomes pregnant, she has a 25 to 30 percent chance of passing her infection on to her baby.

For some time, the U.S. Centers for Disease Control and Prevention (CDC) has been telling us that HIV testing should be a routine part of patient care, pregnant or not. Yet despite this public warning, fewer than half of American adults between 18 and 64 have ever been tested, and only 20 percent have been tested within the last 12 months.

Today, most obstetricians and family doctors are routinely offering HIV testing to pregnant women. It won't hurt for you to be proactive and ask to be tested, whether your doctor offers the test or not.

A further thought: For those pregnant women who do test positive, a medicine called zidovudine (brand name: Retrovir) can reduce the rate of HIV transmission from mother to baby by two-thirds.

Fetal growth and development

"He who sees things from the beginning will have the finest view of them."

Aristotle, 384–322 B.C.

D. Gary Benfield, M.D.

SPERM OR EGG: WHICH ONE DECIDES A BABY'S SEX?

Q *Can you please settle an argument? What determines a baby's sex: The mother's egg or the father's sperm?*

A The human embryo begins to develop at conception or fertilization, when the sperm unites with the ovum or egg to form a single cell called the zygote. The zygote contains 46 chromosomes, 23 from the sperm and 23 from the ovum. As the zygote divides and multiplies into millions of cells, each cell contains a copy of the original 46 chromosomes.

Two of the 46 chromosomes are called sex chromosomes: one from the sperm and one from the ovum. The ovum's chromosome sex is always X, but the sperm's chromosome sex may be X or Y.

Fertilization of the ovum by an X-bearing sperm produces an XX zygote, which normally develops into a female. Fertilization of the ovum by a Y-bearing sperm produces an XY zygote, which normally develops into a male. Thus, the father's sperm—not the mother's ovum—determines a baby's sex.

GESTATIONAL AGE IS NOT THE SAME AS CONCEPTUAL AGE

Q *I'm confused. Can you explain the difference between gestational age and conceptual age when talking about the fetus?*

A When your obstetrician says you're 20 weeks pregnant, he is using gestational age, which is measured from the first day of your last menstrual period **before** conception.

Because the first day of your last menstrual period before conception typically occurs two weeks before conception, gestational age is two weeks longer than conceptual age, which is measured from the day of conception.

So when your obstetrician says you're 20 weeks pregnant, meaning your unborn baby's gestational age is 20 weeks, only 18 weeks have actually gone by since your baby was conceived. By tradition, then, and for no other reason, obstetricians start measuring the length of pregnancy two weeks before conception actually occurs. Confusing? Yes.

A further thought: Your obstetrician and all the pregnancy books will say the typical, full-term pregnancy lasts 40 weeks or 280 days, measured from the first day of your last menstrual period. So the typical full-term baby's gestational age at birth is 40 weeks.

To calculate your due date, then, you can do it by one of two ways:

- Get out your calendar and count 280 days or 40 weeks from the first day of your last menstrual period. Say, for example, the first day of your last menstrual period was January 16, 2006. Then your due date would be October 23, 2006.
- Using the same example, count back three months from January 16 to October 16. Then add seven days. This method will also give you your due date of October 23.

INTRAUTERINE GROWTH RETARDATION

Q *My baby was born full-term, but she only weighed 4 pounds, 6 ounces. She's now three months old, seems healthy, and is growing like a weed. The doctor said she was small because of intrauterine growth retardation. Does that mean she'll likely be mentally retarded? By the way, I'm only five feet, three inches tall and my husband is five foot, seven. So we weren't expecting a big baby anyway. I also smoked about a pack a day during most of my pregnancy.*

A I try to avoid using the term *intrauterine growth retardation* when talking about a baby with her parents. Why? Because it conjures up all kinds of negative images, including one of a mentally retarded child, as it seems to have done for you. Most doctors have switched to calling it intrauterine growth restriction for just that reason.

In your case, your daughter's small size at birth, even though she was full-term, is most likely related to two main factors:

- Your relatively small size
- The fact that you smoked a pack a day during your pregnancy

With good nutrition, most babies born full-term with intrauterine growth restriction catch up with their peers by the end of the first year.
Let your baby's doctor know about your concern. Together, you can keep your eye out for any relatively minor problems, such as hyperactivity or attention-behavioral problems, which sometimes show up later in children born at full-term with intrauterine growth restriction. Also, discuss your concern about mental retardation and confirm my impression that it should not be an issue for your child.

DOES THE FETUS BREATHE IN THE WOMB?

Q *Can you tell me whether the fetus actually breathes inside the womb?*

A The fetus doesn't breathe like you and I do, inhaling oxygen and exhaling carbon dioxide. The baby's mother and the placenta perform those tasks instead. Let me explain.

Oxygen is supplied by mother's oxygen-rich arterial blood, which bathes her side of the placenta. The oxygen then diffuses across the placental membrane and is picked by fetal blood and carried to all parts of the baby's body.

Meanwhile, carbon dioxide travels in the opposite direction, moving across the fetal side of the placenta into mother's circulation. So mom supplies her baby with oxygen and removes her baby's carbon dioxide, all by way of the placenta.

However, the fetus does practice breathing movements. On ultrasound you can see evidence of this activity as small amounts of amniotic fluid move in and out of the lungs.

A further thought: In the seventeenth century, one camp of experts thought each sperm contained a miniature, preformed human being. Another camp thought each ovum contained the same thing. It was not until 1775 that both camps were proven wrong when it was discovered that an ovum and a sperm were necessary to conceive a new human being. So much for expert opinions.

CRITICAL PERIODS OF FETAL DEVELOPMENT

Q *My biology instructor tried to explain why the fetus is more susceptible to the damaging effects of drugs, infectious diseases, and radiation early in pregnancy rather than later. But it was all Greek to me. Can you make it clearer in plain and simple words?*

A It sounds like your instructor was trying to explain the basic concept of "critical periods of development." This term refers to the vulnerability of the developing fetus to damage caused by fetal invaders, such as those you mentioned, at certain time periods during the pregnancy. Why is this idea important? Because it helps us understand how drugs such as cocaine, lithium, thalidomide, and Dilantin, as well as certain viral infections such as German measles, chickenpox, HIV, and others, cross the placenta and invade the developing embryo, causing major birth defects in some fetuses but not in others.

During the first two weeks after conception, if the budding embryo is exposed to certain infectious diseases, drugs, or ionizing radiation, the effect is often fatal, resulting in a miscarriage.

However, during weeks three to nine after conception, a similar invasion may only damage one or more organs, causing one or more birth defects, but not ending the pregnancy. This period in development is a "highly sensitive period" when major defects may be produced.

In general, following this highly sensitive period, a similar invasion will not leave a major defect in its wake because most organs are fully developed by then and only have to grow and mature until birth. However, each organ develops and matures at its own rate, so each organ has its own highly sensitive period as follows:

Highly Sensitive Periods
(weeks after conception)

- Nervous system, Weeks 3 to 16
- Heart, Weeks 3 to 7
- Upper limbs, Weeks 4 to 6
- Eyes, Weeks 4 to 8
- Lower limbs, Weeks 4 to 6
- Teeth, Weeks 6 to 9
- Palate, Weeks 6 to 9
- Genitalia, Weeks 7 to 10
- Ear, Weeks 4 to 9

A further thought: Here are two sample cases to show how we might apply the concept of critical periods of development.

Case #1:

A woman, who is 24 weeks pregnant (22 weeks since conception), was injured in an auto accident. Her full-term baby was born 16 weeks later and found to have a major heart defect. Despite emergency surgery to try and fix the baby's heart problem, the baby died several hours after surgery.

The mother sued the driver of the car that caused the accident for wrongful death, claiming the accident caused her baby's fatal heart defect. Does she have a case?

Because the accident occurred 22 weeks after conception, and because the heart's most sensitive period for an outside factor to cause a defect ends at seven weeks after conception, which means the heart was fully formed long before 22 weeks after conception when the accident occurred, the mother doesn't have a case.

Case #2:

A woman comes down with chickenpox during her seventh week of pregnancy (five weeks after conception). Later, her full-term baby is born with a withered left arm, three stubs for fingers on her left hand, and scarring over the left side of her chest. Is it possible her baby's birth defects were caused by the chickenpox virus?

There is convincing evidence that a maternal chickenpox infection that occurs during the critical period of development for fetal limbs (four to six weeks after conception) has about a 20 percent chance of causing defects involving the limbs, skin scarring, and mental retardation. So yes, it's possible.

D. Gary Benfield, M.D.

Childbirth

ELECTIVE C-SECTION OR VAGINAL DELIVERY: WHICH GAMBLE SHOULD YOU TAKE?

Q *I'm 32 years old, happily married, and 13 weeks along in my first pregnancy. I'm also seriously considering having my baby by elective C-section. Seven months ago, my best friend had her first baby the same way. She says it was really great planning the C-section and not having hours of painful labor. She also says she's planning on one more baby and will not even consider a vaginal birth.*

My husband says it's up to me, but he worries about me having surgery and something going wrong. One of his co-workers shares his concerns. He told my husband that his wife, a mother of three, has had two vaginal births and a C-section. She says it took her twice as long to recover from the C-section than from her vaginal births. I would like to hear your choice since you're a neonatologist. Can you tell me what you think?

A Kenny Rogers, the singer, had a big country-western hit called "The Gambler." The lines that made the song famous go like this:

> You got to know when to hold 'em, know when to fold 'em.
> Know when to walk away and know when to run.

You've been dealt a pretty good hand. You're apparently healthy, only 32, happily married, and going to have your first baby. So far, it's like holding a pair of aces and a pair of kings, a combination that wins most hands. You only need one more ace or one more king to have a sure winner. It's called a full house.

The song continues:

Walking the Baby Beat

> Now every gambler knows that the secret to survivin'
> is knowin' what to throw away and knowin' what to keep.

Hmmm.

You certainly don't want to throw away any of the cards you've been dealt so far, right?

You just need one more card to complete the hand and give you the very best chance of winning.

What's that card? A healthy baby and a healthy mom *after* you've given birth, that other ace or king for sure.

So which way of giving birth gives you the best chance of drawing that final ace or king: a spontaneous vaginal delivery or a planned C-section?

As you probably know, a growing number of C-sections are elective, meaning they're done at mom's request for one or more of the following reasons:

- I want to decide when my baby will deliver.
- I want to fit my baby's birth into my career.
- I want to have a sense of control over my body.
- I want to be sure to have the doctor of my choice.
- I want to know that my husband and family will be there for support.
- I want to be free of pain.
- I want to protect my vagina and not risk later incontinence.
- I want to protect my baby and not risk a loss of oxygen to his brain or through the use of forceps.

Notice how only one of the reasons on this list has anything to do with having a healthy baby. Notice also how all of those reasons overlook the following facts:

- A C-section is major abdominal surgery.
- A C-section carries the risk of bleeding and infection.
- A C-section carries the risk that something may go wrong with anesthesia.

- A C-section carries the risk of temporary breathing problems for the baby, due to excess fluid remaining in the lungs.
- A C-section carries the risk of more serious respiratory problems for the baby, due to lung immaturity.
- A C-section probably means "Once a section, always a section," because fewer and fewer doctors are allowing vaginal delivery after a previous section, due to the risk of rupturing the uterus.
- A C-section carries the risk of later adhesions, causing twisting and pulling in the abdomen, possibly leading to infertility, pelvic pain, and bowel obstruction.
- A C-section carries the risk of having to use a suction device applied to the baby's head to help remove her from the uterus. (Not all babies can be removed from the uterus simply by hand.)

What do I think? I think your best chance of having a healthy baby and a healthy mom *after* you've given birth is to hold the cards Mother Nature dealt you so far and trust her to deal you that final ace or king by having a vaginal delivery. If things change, even at the last minute, you can still win the hand by having a C-section.

For more insight into this issue, read the next question and answer.

SOME BABIES TAKE LONGER TO ADJUST AT BIRTH

Q *Our daughter was born three weeks ago by planned cesarean because my wife didn't want to go through labor. The baby weighed 7 pounds and 3 ounces and had two problems: She breathed faster than normal for about 24 hours and her blood glucose was low for about 8 hours. The pediatrician* *said something about extra fluid in her lungs. He also said this condition was temporary, and he was right. My wife and daughter came home together five days after birth. Based on what I've told you, can you explain why our daughter had problems? So far, she's doing fine at home.*

A Let's think about what happened this way. Before birth, your daughter received a continuous flow of glucose, oxygen, and other nutrients from your wife through the placenta. Your wife also kept the baby warm.

At the moment of birth, your baby rapidly changed or transitioned from total dependence on her mom to limited independence. For most babies, this transition period goes smoothly: They breathe on their own, cry within seconds, and begin controlling their own glucose level and body temperature, as long as they're dried off and wrapped in a blanket. In fact, most babies can be put to breast within the first hour after birth. However, for a few babies, like your daughter, this transition period takes longer.

Let's talk about the breathing problem first. At the moment of birth, all babies have some fluid left in their lungs, especially those babies delivered by elective cesarean section without going through labor. The process of labor normally squeezes up to two-thirds of the lung fluid out of the lungs by the moment of birth. Think of each contraction as preparing the lungs for the first breath.

In your daughter's case, her lungs were still full of fluid at birth, because she hadn't experienced those contractions. The larger the amount of fluid left in the lungs, the greater the effort it takes to breathe. So the baby breathes faster than normal until her body reabsorbs the remaining lung fluid. This process may take several hours to several days. It represents a delay in transition, not a disease.

Now, let's move on to the glucose issue. At birth, the continuous flow of glucose from mother to the baby is interrupted. Now the baby must regulate her own glucose level while she adjusts to being fed every few hours.

The resulting blood glucose level depends on a fine balance between several factors:

- Frequency and volume of milk intake
- Glucose production by the liver
- The amount of insulin produced by the pancreas

Too much insulin, too little milk intake, or decreased glucose production can each contribute to a low blood sugar.

Usually, the baby herself makes these adjustments. Occasionally, when a full-term baby is breathing too fast to suck, intravenous glucose is needed temporarily until the baby settles down. That apparently wasn't necessary in your daughter's case. She was able to raise her blood glucose level on her own.

It sounds like your baby's problems are over and done with.

Congratulations!

A further thought: An increasing number of women are having their babies by elective cesarean section rather than letting nature take its course and going through labor. This case illustrates what can happen when a baby is delivered by elective section with its lungs still full of fluid. Though this baby's problems were relatively mild, some babies have even required intensive care for breathing problems after an elective section. Expectant mothers need to know of this possibility before making an informed decision to have an elective cesarean birth.

WHAT IS A DOULA?

Q *During my last childbirth class, the instructor mentioned that more and more expectant parents are hiring a specially* *trained person to help them with their births. Can you tell me what she was talking about? What does this person do?*

A Your instructor was probably referring to a *doula*, a Greek word that has come to mean "the woman who mothers the mother during her labor and birth experience." Once labor begins, the doula provides continuous emotional, physical, and educational support for her laboring patient and the baby's father. She can also help them write a birth plan.

Some doulas are childbirth educators while others are registered nurses. All have years of experience before becoming certified.

Recent research has shown the following impressive benefits for mothers who have the continuous support of a doula during labor and birth:

- Shortens first-time labor by an average of 25 percent
- Reduces the need for a cesarean section by 50 percent
- Reduces the use of drugs to stimulate labor by 40 percent
- Reduces requests for epidural anesthesia by 60 percent
- Reduces the need for forceps-assisted birth by 40 percent

Doula-assisted mothers described their labors and births as less painful; they felt more in control of birth; and they felt less anxious after birth. Also, their babies had fewer complications and fewer health problems at the six week checkup.

On the other hand, the most difficult situation a pregnant couple will ever face occurs when they learn that their unborn baby has a fatal birth defect and will only live a short time after the baby is born. Here are excerpts from an actual birth plan that a doula helped such a couple prepare:

- After birth we would like to assist with David's footprints.
- If David has a sucking instinct, Carolyn would like to nurse him. Even if he's not actively sucking, she would like to hold him close to her breast.
- We want as many memories of David as possible and for that reason will have pictures taken when he is born.
- We understand that you will prepare a memory folder for us with David's footprints, photo, and a lock of his hair.
- Carolyn has made a special hat for David for his memory folder picture. Please remind us to put it on him if we forget.
- We will be bringing Holy water in a special little cup for David's baptism. If our pastor is present he will baptize David. If not, we will do it ourselves.
- We would like to remain together as a family in the postpartum room on OB.
- If David should live past the days Carolyn needs to remain in the hospital, we want to consider taking him home with us. We have arranged a strong family support system for possible short-term home care.
- We have made arrangements with _____ funeral home to care for David when he goes home to be with the Lord. Our contact person there is _____.
- We have discussed an autopsy and have decided to _____.

If you would like to learn more about what doulas have to offer, you can ask your childbirth instructor or call Doulas of North America at 206-324-5440 in Seattle, Washington.

IS LABOR LONGER FOR WOMEN WHO DELIVER BOYS?

Q *My mother says that labor takes longer for women who give birth to boys than it does for women who give birth to girls. Is this true?*

A Yes. Studies have shown that the average length of labor for women delivering boys is about one hour longer than that for women delivering girls.

ANTICIPATING PROBLEMS AT BIRTH IS GOOD CARE

Q *I am expecting the birth of twin girls at the end of December, and everything has gone great so far. My OB says a nurse will be assigned to each baby just in case they need help in the delivery room. My husband and I appreciate the thought, but is it really necessary?*

A Here is the universal standard of care that exists in every hospital that provides obstetrical services:

- One person, who is skilled in resuscitating the baby and whose sole responsibility is the baby, must be present at every delivery.
- To avoid any delays, the equipment and supplies necessary to perform a complete resuscitation must also be available at every delivery.
- When twins or higher multiples are involved, each baby is entitled to its own caregiver and its own equipment.

Is all this really necessary?
Studies show that from 3 to 7 percent of all newborns require some form of resuscitation at birth. The odds of

this happening increase somewhat when twins or higher multiples are involved.

I'm not trying to cast a cloud over your pregnancy, but unexpected problems can occur right up to the last minute of labor and delivery. If a baby is born who won't breathe or is having difficulty breathing, and no one is in charge of the baby, and no one knows where the resuscitation equipment is or how to use it, the resulting chaotic response can lead to a nightmare of the worst kind.

Anticipating problems and being prepared is the cornerstone of good delivery room care.

EMERGENCY CHILDBIRTH CAN HAPPEN TO ANYONE

Q *I'm six months pregnant, and my husband travels a lot. What should I do if I am home alone, go into labor, and can't make it to the hospital?*

A Emergency childbirth can happen to anyone, so the best thing to do is be prepared.

Make sure you have the names and telephone numbers of your doctor, the hospital where you plan to deliver, and nearby family or friends written down and near the phone.

If you feel what you think is the onset of labor or your water breaks, remember these guidelines:

- Call your doctor or the obstetrical unit in the hospital where you plan to deliver for advice.
- Call a neighbor or a family member for help.
- If you are having frequent contractions, call 9-1-1.
- Try not to push or bear down.
- Find a comfortable place, and spread out towels or blankets.
- If the baby comes before help arrives, try to use your hands to ease the baby out while you gently push.

- Wrap the baby in a clean towel or blanket.
- Use a clean wash cloth or tissue to remove mucus from the baby's mouth.
- Do not pull on the umbilical cord to deliver the placenta. It usually slides out within five to ten minutes.
- Once it delivers, keep the placenta at the level of the baby, not below it.
- You don't need to cut the cord.
- Hold your snugly wrapped baby close to your body to keep it warm until help arrives.

A further thought: If you unexpectedly give birth at home, you should still let someone take you and your baby to the hospital to be checked and observed for at least 24 hours.

SIGNS OF BIRTH INJURY MAY NOT SHOW UP RIGHT AWAY

Q *Our first child, Laura, was born almost five weeks ago by natural childbirth. It was the most moving experience of my life. And certainly Laura was the most perfect baby I had ever seen. But when I took her in for her two-week checkup, our pediatrician noticed a lump near Laura's shoulder. She said it was probably a broken collar bone that had already started to heal. She sent us for X-rays which confirmed her diagnosis. Can you tell me how such an easy birth could break her collar bone? Could someone have mishandled my precious baby and broken the bone by mistake?*

A Take a deep breath and relax. Medically speaking, your daughter, Laura, sustained a fractured clavicle, otherwise known as the collar bone. (Incidentally, the clavicle is fractured more often than any other bone during the newborn period.)

Most clavicle fractures occur when the head and shoulders are forcefully manipulated during a difficult birth. It's sometimes the price we pay for delivering the baby safely. However, the clavicle may also fracture during a relatively easy birth, such as yours. It all depends on the forces of labor, the anatomy of the mother's pelvis, and the position of the baby during labor and delivery.

Apparently, your daughter's fractured clavicle wasn't noticed in the nursery, and you didn't notice anything out of the ordinary after you took her home. Why? Because she wasn't in pain, which might have caused her to limit her arm movement on the affected side and draw attention to the problem.

Meanwhile, the bone started to heal by forming a callus at the fracture site. This overgrowth of bone was the lump your doctor noticed at Laura's two-week checkup.

Sometimes the diagnosis of a fractured clavicle in the newborn period is not made until months or even years later when an X-ray taken for some other purpose surprisingly reveals callus formation at an old fracture site. Regardless of when a fractured clavicle is diagnosed, the treatment is usually the same: watchful waiting.

Some parents tend to blame the medical staff when something goes wrong in childbirth, especially when it adversely affects the baby. I seriously doubt that anyone involved in your daughter's care did anything to cause her fracture. As for Laura, it sounds like her clavicle is healing nicely.

A further thought: Toddlers just starting to walk frequently fall. After a fall, they often limp for a few hours. Any toddler who limps longer than 24 hours deserves medical attention to rule out a bone fracture or an injury to the hip joint.

USING A SUCTION CUP TO COMPLETE DELIVERY

Q *Shortly after our daughter was born, my wife and I noticed her head was swollen and bruised. The nurse said it* was caused by a suction cup the doctor had attached to the baby's head to help complete the delivery.

It took several weeks for the swelling to go down and the bruise to disappear. Our pediatrician even checked the baby's blood count to make sure she hadn't lost too much blood in her scalp. Can you tell me if this rather brutal way of delivering babies is common practice? Is it safe?

A Applying suction to a baby's scalp to help complete certain deliveries has replaced the use of forceps in many hospitals around the country. Studies comparing forceps with suction have not shown a significant difference in success rate or complications. Thus, the choice of instrument frequently comes down to doctor preference.

A further thought: Like any other medical treatment, these suction devices should only be used when the benefits clearly outweigh the risks. Expectant mothers should discuss this issue with their doctor before their baby is born.

WRITING A BIRTH PLAN

Q *I'm 24 weeks pregnant with my first child. My husband and I would like to have some say in what happens when I go into labor and the actual birth itself. But my doctor is so busy that I haven't been able to tell her how I feel about these issues. Can you offer any suggestions?*

A One solution to your problem is to write out a birth plan. A birth plan is simply a written description of your priorities and preferred choices during labor and birth and afterward. The plan can be placed in your chart, where those involved in your care can read it. The part that pertains to your baby (the baby care plan) can be placed in your baby's chart, which is usually separate from your own.

Writing a birth plan offers several advantages:

- Simply preparing the plan will help you focus on various choices. For example, natural versus medicated childbirth, circumcision versus no circumcision, breastfeeding versus bottle feeding.
- It encourages you and your husband to discuss your worries and expectations, and to come to some agreement on what is most important.
- You don't have to take the time and trouble to tell each staff member your wishes on every choice as they come up during your labor.
- A birth plan also helps your doctor. If you prepare a rough draft and go over it with her, she will learn more about you as well as your preferences and will know how to help you in labor. She can also help you modify your choices that may seem unwise or inappropriate.

You might begin your birth plan by simply stating that you appreciate the staff's help and advice. Then you might describe yourself and anything you feel would help the staff understand you and your birth plan better.

For example, if you experienced a long period of infertility, or if you had unpleasant experiences in hospitals in the past, tell them. If a natural birth is important to you, let them know so they can offer you the kind of support you will need.

In the next part of your birth plan simply list your preferences about common procedures that are often optional if all is going well. These procedures include the following:

- An enema in early labor
- The use of intravenous fluids
- Electronic fetal monitoring
- Breaking the bag of waters
- Pain medication and restriction to bed

Baby preferences might address the following choices:

- Ways for keeping your baby warm
- Putting your baby to breast
- Spending time with your baby
- Circumcision, if it's a boy

Your birth plan should be flexible, taking into account not only an ideal labor but also the possibility of a difficult labor or other unexpected events.

At the moment, you may feel like you don't have enough background to decide your preferences about some of these issues. Childbirth classes, discussions with your doctor, and books, such as *Your Pregnancy: Questions and Answers* by Glade B. Curtis, M.D., are helpful resources.

DID MY PEDIATRICIAN CHARGE TOO MUCH?

Q *My baby was born at 5:10 in the morning, and we both went home the next day. Since I was taking insulin for diabetes and considered high risk, my pediatrician, who lives 20 minutes from the hospital, was called to come in for my delivery. After examining the baby and checking his blood sugar, she assured me everything was all right. The following day, she reexamined the baby and said he was ready for discharge. Later, she sent me a bill for $105. This amount seems rather steep to me, but I want to be fair. Can you tell me if she charged too much?*

A Let's see if I've got the facts straight. Your pediatrician was called out of bed in the middle of the night to attend your baby's birth. She got dressed and drove 20 minutes to the hospital. She probably reviewed your medical history, noting any risk factors that might affect your baby, and checked the resuscitation equipment to make sure everything was ready in case your baby had a problem.

D. Gary Benfield, M.D.

Once your baby was born, she probably helped dry off your baby under an overhead heater and sucked out any excess mucus from his nose and throat. Then, she examined him from head to toe, looking for signs of a low blood sugar, difficulty breathing, and any evidence of birth defects. (These symptoms all occur more frequently in infants of diabetic mothers.)

She ordered a blood sugar, checked the results, then reassured you that everything was all right. She probably arrived back home just in time to get ready for another day at the office.

The following day, she returned to the hospital, checked on his progress, examined the baby, and stopped by your room to discuss plans for discharge and follow-up at her office.

Seems to me, you got a bargain. Suppose, during that first hour or so, your baby had developed seizures caused by a low blood sugar. She was there to prevent that from happening. Or, suppose your baby had difficulty breathing and needed life-saving resuscitation. She was there to intervene if necessary.

In addition, she returned the next day, checked on his progress, and went over discharge plans. I suggest you consider the following:

- Send her a check for $105.00 and enclose a thank-you note.
- Then, tell all your friends about this wonderful pediatrician who went out of her way, in the middle of the night, to help your baby get off to a good start.

A further thought: It was 1902 when Morris Mitchtom named a stuffed little bear the "Teddy Bear" in honor of Theodore Roosevelt after reading that T. R. refused to shoot a captured cub on a hunting trip.

ALL YOU EVER WANTED TO KNOW ABOUT CESAREAN BIRTH

Q *I'm almost eight months pregnant with my first baby and planning for a vaginal birth. Just in case, can you explain how a cesarean section is done and the different circumstances that might make a cesarean birth necessary?*

A It's probably a good idea to educate yourself about cesarean birth because most first-time cesareans occur unexpectedly. Without going into too much detail, a cesarean section involves the following steps:

- The surgeon makes the initial incision through the skin in the middle of the mother's lower abdomen, then he extends the incision deeper through the muscles that make up the abdominal wall, exposing the uterus.
- He then makes an incision through the muscular wall of the uterus, being careful to avoid damaging the urinary bladder nearby. Now he can see the fetus within the sac that also contains your amniotic fluid.
- Occasionally, the surgeon may encounter the placenta when he cuts through the uterus. He can simply cut through the placenta, which increases the risk of fetal blood loss due to hemorrhage, or he can modify his incision and try to avoid the placenta.
- As soon as the surgeon cuts open the amniotic sac, a gush of fluid fills his field of view. He inserts his hand into the uterine cavity and raises the baby's head through the uterine incision. As soon as the baby's head is completely delivered, the surgeon suctions the baby's mouth and nose to clear the airway of fluid and mucus. An assistant then applies

pressure to the mother's lower abdomen, forcing delivery of the rest of the baby.
- The surgeon then applies two clamps to the baby's umbilical cord and cuts the cord between the two clamps.
- The baby is then handed off to a nurse who places the baby on an open bed, located under an overhead warmer.
- Following delivery of the baby, the placenta starts to detach from the inner wall of the uterus and usually delivers spontaneously within minutes after the baby is born.
- After inspecting the uterine cavity for any residual bleeding, the surgeon closes the uterine incision, then the abdominal wall incision, and then the skin, all with sutures.
- However, before closing the abdominal wall, the surgeon examines the uterus, fallopian tubes and ovaries for any unsuspected problems.

A cesarean birth might be necessary for one of the following reasons:

- Your labor fails to progress normally or stops altogether. This situation is one of the most common reasons that doctors deliver babies by cesarean.
- Your baby has an abnormal heart rate pattern during labor, indicting a problem with the baby's oxygen supply.
- Your baby is in an abnormal position, such as feet first, buttocks first, or in a transverse position.
- You have a serious medical problem. If you have diabetes, heart disease, lung disease, or high blood pressure, you may need a cesarean birth. Also, if you have a vaginal herpes simplex infection, you may need a cesarean to avoid exposing the baby to this serious disease during vaginal delivery.

Walking the Baby Beat

- You are carrying twins, triplets, or higher multiples. About half of all women who have twins have cesarean births. Triplets and higher multiples are another story. More than 90 percent of triplets and higher multiples are delivered by cesarean section.
- A problem develops with your placenta. In one instance, the placenta starts to detach too soon from the inner wall of your uterus, which can be life-threatening for you and your baby. In the second instance, your placenta is implanted low in your uterus and partially or completely covers the opening of your cervix. Women with both of these placental problems usually have a cesarean section
- There's a problem with the umbilical cord. Once your water has broken, a loop of cord may slip out through your cervix, ahead of the baby. As your baby presses against the cervix, pressure on the protruding cord may block your baby's oxygen supply, forcing your doctor to do an immediate cesarean section.
- Your baby is very large. Some babies are just too large to deliver safely vaginally, especially if you have a small pelvis, which may prevent the baby's head from passing through.

A further thought: A cesarean birth is major surgery. It carries certain risks, including the risk of death. The risk of death following a cesarean birth is estimated at two in 10,000, about twice the risk of a vaginal birth.

DELIVERY ROOM MOTTO: BE PREPARED!

One morning a few years ago, I had just finished making rounds in the nursery when Cindy Goldman, the head nurse in OB, stopped me in the hall.

"Dr. Crawford has a patient in labor who's bleeding, complete, and pushing," she said. "I'm worried about the baby. But ole Crawford's too stubborn to ask for help. Would you do me a favor and stand by, just in case?"

As head nurses go, Cindy really knew her stuff. If she was worried about a baby, I had better listen. So I headed over to labor and delivery, put on a gown, and slipped inside the delivery room.

Crawford was perched on a stool at the foot of the bed, waiting for the next contraction. I could see the baby's head on the perineum. One more push should do it.

"Out looking for business?" Crawford asked, staring straight ahead.

"No sir," I said. "Just watching a master at work."

His patient lay flat on her back, panting through partly-open lips. "Please God, save my baby," she prayed. Then she arched her back, let out a scream, and pushed out her baby into Crawford's waiting hands.

The little girl was silent, limp, and blue.

Crawford cradled the baby in one hand and suctioned bloody mucus from the mouth and nose with the other. Then he clamped the cord, cut it with scissors, and handed her off to Jodi Bailey, the nurse assigned to the baby.

Jodi placed the child under the overhead warmer, wiped her off with a warm blanket, and suctioned her mouth and nose again.

I slipped on a pair of gloves, grabbed a stethoscope, and moved in to help. Jodi rubbed the baby's back, trying to get her to breathe, while I listened to her heart and lungs.

At birth, a baby's heart usually beats between 120 and 140 times per minute, twice as fast as most adults. But I only counted 80. And she still hadn't taken her first breath.

When a baby is deprived of oxygen, it reacts in a predictable way. First, the heart's pumping action weakens, accounting for the slow pulse. Then the flow of blood to all the organs is diverted to the brain and heart to support their vital functions.

We had three minutes to start breathing for the baby and to strengthen the heart's pumping action before she might suffer brain damage and multiple organ failure. Her life hung in the balance.

Fortunately, Jodi had already laid out the resuscitation equipment and checked it over, just in case. So everything was ready.

I flipped open the blade on a laryngoscope and slid it over the baby's tongue to visualize her airway. Then I slid a breathing tube down into her trachea. We attached the tube to a breathing bag and started ventilating the baby, using 100 percent oxygen.

"Good breath sounds on both sides," Jodi said, as she listened through the rise and fall of the baby's chest with her stethoscope. "Heart rate's picking up, now above 100."

The baby's color changed from blue to pink. Then she started moving her arms and legs.

Suddenly, and without any warning, she spit out the tube in protest, as if to say, "I'm ready to breathe on my own, thank you." Like beautiful music, her uncontrolled crying filled the room.

I glanced over at her mother. She was propped up on her elbows, looking toward the delicious sound and smiling. Her prayers had been answered, thanks to Cindy Goldman and Jodi Bailey, who prepared ahead of time, before action was really needed.

A further thought: The names of persons mentioned in this story have been changed from the names of those actually present at the delivery.

THE CESAREAN SECTION RATE KEEPS GOING UP

Talking to myself about the cesarean-section rate in this country:

I: If I were to ask you how often women in this country give birth by cesarean section, what would you guess?
Me: Five percent of all births.
I: Higher.
Me: Ten percent?
I: Nope, too low.
Me: Fifteen percent?
I: Still too low.
Me: How about 20 percent?
I: Not even close.
Me: Alright, already! What's the answer?
I: It will surprise you.
Me: Look knucklehead, quit playing games!
I: C'mon, take another guess.
Me: Not on your life! What's the answer?
I: The cesarean delivery rate in 2002 was 26.1 percent, the highest ever recorded.
Me: Are you kidding? That's one in every four births.
I: I always knew you were good at math.
Me: Cut the sarcasm, okay?
I: Sorry.
Me: So why so many sections?
I: For one thing, the primary cesarean rate, that's the number of women having a section for the first time, keeps going up. Another thing is the sharp decline in the number of women giving birth vaginally after a previous section.
Me: Why is that?
I: Some experts say a vaginal birth after a previous cesarean isn't safe for mom or for baby.
Me: So we're back to the old adage, "Once a cesarean, always a cesarean."
I: Close to it.

Walking the Baby Beat

Me: Say, remember 20 or 25 years ago when the section rate at each of the area hospitals was less than 10 percent?

I: Sure do. In fact, the hospitals used to compare each other's monthly statistics to see who had the lowest rate.

Me: Remember what would happen if the monthly cesarean rate climbed higher than 10 percent?

I: Yep. The Chief of OB would stand up at the monthly department meeting, get a stern look on his face, and shake his finger at the medical staff. "Boys and girls," he would say, "you're doing too many unnecessary sections. That's bad practice!" You could hear a pin drop.

Me: Of course, he also said it was bad practice when women started asking if their husbands could be with them in the delivery room. But that's another story.

I: So what's changed?

Me: We could blame it on the lawyers.

I: What do you mean by that?

Me: Obstetricians today are forced to practice defensive medicine and do more cesareans. Otherwise, if they get a damaged baby and didn't do a section, they're more likely to get sued.

I: What else has changed?

Me: Believe it or not, more and more women are demanding elective cesarean births, something that would have been unthinkable 20 or 30 years ago.

I: That's crazy! Don't they know a cesarean is major surgery?

Me: Quiet. Let's not go there.

I: What do you see for the future?

Me: I think the national C-section rate will keep inching up. What's to stop it?

D. Gary Benfield, M.D.

WATER BIRTH: DANGEROUS FAD OR EMPOWERING RITUAL?

It was no accident that Cathie gave birth in a portable pool. She and her partner, Laurens, planned it that way as part of an elaborate birthing plan she had typed up and discussed with her certified nurse-midwife, Barbara Harper, months before giving birth.

But what surprised even Harper, who has assisted with many water births, was Cathie's plan to deliver in Barbados. This meant shipping a portable birthing pool by boat from Miami to Barbados where the couple turned their veranda into a cozy birthing room.

Cathie labored most of the night. As her labor grew more intense, she and her partner entered the pool, which was heated to 98 degrees. Laurens rubbed Cathie's back and hips, as directed by Harper, until, according to plan, baby Phoenix was born under water, weighing 8 pounds, 12 ounces.

"I would definitely do the water birth again," said Cathie.

But not every birthing plan that calls for a water birth ends like Cathie's, according to a study published in *Pediatrics*, the medical journal of the American Academy of Pediatrics.

The study involved four full-term newborns who were transferred, over an 18-month period, to a neonatal intensive care unit in Auckland, New Zealand, after delivering under water at other hospitals.

- Each of the four babies had chest X-rays and clinical findings consistent with a near-drowning experience.
- All required respirator support, the longest for three days.
- One was readmitted at nine days of age with seizures. Tests of brain function turned out to be

normal, and no additional seizures occurred in the hospital. The child's development at one year of age was normal.
- The other three infants did well after going home.

Dr. Ruth Gilbert, a physician at the Institute of Health in London, discussed the pros and cons of water birth in a separate article that also appeared in the same issue of *Pediatrics*.

Can delivery in water cause serious adverse outcomes? "Undoubtedly, the answer is yes," said Gilbert.

As warning, she cited several reports of death attributable to drowning as a result of poorly managed water births.

One death, involving two experienced midwives, was caused by asphyxiation and water-logged lungs, which made resuscitation of the infant difficult, said Gilbert. As a result of that case, water births have been banned in Sweden.

Some women are prepared to trade off a presumably small risk of a very serious outcome against the perceived benefits for the infant and the mother who has a water birth.

But there is no clear research evidence that immersion in water during labor reduces duration of labor, perineal tears, or the use of analgesia, according to Gilbert. Additionally, data comparing the risk of water birth to that of low-risk nonwater births are not available.

Advocates of water birth believe pregnant women have the right to choose between water birth and more mainstream approaches to giving birth. But these same advocates also have the responsibility to provide balanced information, including the potential harms of water birth.

For couples who are still curious and want more information about water birth, see Barbara Harper's Web site at www.waterbirth.org.

WHAT HAPPENS IF MY PREGNANCY GOES TOO LONG?

Q *I know that premature birth can be dangerous for the baby. But what if my pregnancy lasts longer than nine months?*

A A pregnancy is considered overdue or postterm when it exceeds 41 completed weeks (full term is 40 weeks, plus or minus two weeks). This happens in about 10 percent of all pregnancies.

The majority of babies born two or more weeks past their due date are delivered safely. However, you have to remember the placenta is aging too. This may mean the placenta is reaching the point where it will no longer be able to continuously provide an adequate supply of oxygen and nutrients to meet a postmature baby's needs.

Depending on the results of one or more special tests of fetal well-being, the doctor may intervene when a pregnancy exceeds 41 completed weeks by inducing labor, using intravenous Pitocin. If the baby shows signs of distress, a doctor may recommend performing a cesarean section.

Storing cord blood

STORING CORD BLOOD OFFERS PEACE OF MIND, AT A PRICE

Q *I'm seven and a half months pregnant for the first time. My husband and I have talked about possibly saving our baby's cord blood just in case the baby might need it in the future. But we haven't discussed it with my doctor. Do you think this idea is goofy or something worth pursuing? Do you know how much it costs?*

A Let's back up a bit and explain some things about fetal blood so we can better understand what you are talking about.

Before birth, the fetal heart pumps blood throughout its circulation, just like you and me. But unlike you and me, the blood also flows through the umbilical cord to the placenta, where it picks up oxygen and other nutrients and then returns to the heart. This continuous flow of blood throughout the fetal circulation persists right up to the moment of birth, before the cord is clamped.

All of this fetal blood is rich in fetal stem cells, which have the potential to heal certain diseases and repair certain tissues. (In contrast, that tiny ball of embryonic stem cells, which implanted in the wall of the uterus and grew over a period of nine months to become this baby, were totipotent, meaning they had the potential to become any organ or tissue within the baby.)

At birth, after the umbilical cord is clamped and cut, several ounces of fetal blood remain behind within the fetal side of the placenta and the part of the cord that is still attached to the placenta. It is this cord blood you may decide to have collected and stored for possible future use.

In order to decide whether your idea is goofy or worthwhile, let's ask two questions:

- **First, what are the odds that your baby or another family member might ever need the fetal stem cells in the stored blood?**

According to medical research, the odds that a child will need to use her own cord blood stem cells for one of the 75 diseases that have already been successfully treated with stem cells are 1 in 2,700. The odds that another family member might need to use those cells are about 1 in 1,400. So for every 2,700 families that store their baby's cord blood, one child and two family members might use it. Put differently, 2,697 families will *not need* it for their child or a family member. Of course, those odds may improve over time as medical science increases the number of diseases successfully treated with stored fetal stem cells.

- **Second, what does it cost to collect your baby's cord blood and store it?**

According to Cord Blood Registry, the largest provider of stored cord blood services, the company charges a one-time payment fee of $1,975 for a collection kit, shipping, processing, and testing, and the first year of storage. For storing the blood until the age of 18, the company charges a fixed annual fee of $125 per year, beginning with the second year of storage. However, if you pay the entire 18-year storage fee in advance, you can save $400 on the 18-year storage fee, for a total cost of $3,700. This payment is due after the sample has been processed and stored. If you are unable to pay up front, the company has payment plans that will increase the total cost to slightly more than $4,000.

- **So the question becomes, is it worth roughly $4,000 to collect and store your baby's cord blood for 18 years when the chances of that blood being needed for your child or a family member is currently 3 in 2,700, or 1 in 900?**

According to Cord Blood Registry's Web site (www.cordblood.com), the company has stored more than 270,000 units of cord blood. Those families, then, have answered our question with a resounding yes; it's worth it to them. Their total cost, including 18 years of storage: More than $1.1 billion.

- **Do I think it's a goofy idea or something worth pursuing?**

It seems worth pursuing if you can afford it, and it gives you peace of mind.

On the other hand, if you go ahead and add 60 monthly payments plus annual storage fees to your maxed-out credit card debt, your monthly car payment, and your monthly mortgage payment, then, yes, it's probably a goofy idea.

A further thought: Cord blood transplants started in 1990 when Mathew Farrow, then age 6, received the first cord-blood transfusion or transplant, using cord blood from his newly born sister. Mathew suffered from Fanconi's Anemia, a genetic blood disease that usually kills its victims by the age of 12.

Unable to find a matching bone marrow donor, Mathew's parents flew him to Paris, France, where Mathew received a transfusion of his sister's cord blood. Now, 15 years later, Mathew is alive and healthy, and cord blood transplantation has spread worldwide.

Premature baby care

IF JACKIE KENNEDY'S PREMATURE SON, PATRICK, WERE BORN TODAY, WOULD HE SURVIVE?

Q *If I remember correctly, didn't Jackie Kennedy have two premature sons: John, Jr. who later died in a plane crash in 1999, and Patrick, who died shortly after birth in 1963? If Patrick were born today, what would his chances be of surviving?*

A Your memory serves you well. John Jr. was born four weeks early by emergency cesarean section on November 25, 1960, at Georgetown University Hospital in Washington, D.C. He weighed 6 pounds, 3 ounces, stayed in an incubator for five days, and was discharged in good health at two weeks of age. (Six weeks later, his father was inaugurated president of the United States.)

Patrick was born five-and-a-half weeks early by emergency cesarean section on August 7, 1963, at Otis Air Force Base Hospital on Cape Cod. Weighing 4 pounds, 10 ounces, he had difficulty breathing and was rushed by ambulance to Children's Hospital in Boston.

Despite receiving the best of care, Patrick died 40 hours after birth from hyaline membrane disease, a common breathing problem of premature infants caused by underdeveloped lungs. (Fifteen weeks later, on November 22, his father was assassinated in Dallas, Texas.)

Stimulated in part by Patrick Kennedy's highly publicized death from hyaline membrane disease, obstetricians and pediatricians in this country began working closer together in the late 1960s to improve the outcome of pregnancy. As a result, medicine today has a lot more to offer pregnant women like Jacqueline Kennedy and premature babies like Patrick. For example:

- Obstetricians who specialize in problem pregnancies (perinatologists) and pediatricians who specialize in caring for sick newborns (neonatologists) can be found in most large cities.
- Drugs are now available to stop premature labor, speed up fetal lung development, and help prevent hyaline membrane disease, the breathing problem that took Patrick Kennedy's short life.
- Thanks to these and other advances, babies born five to six weeks early like Patrick usually do well and grow up as healthy children.

A further thought: Jacqueline Kennedy never again saw Patrick after he was rushed to Boston. While she recovered from her cesarean birth in the hospital on Cape Cod, Patrick's funeral mass and burial were held in Boston, attended by her husband, President Kennedy, and a few family friends. In effect, she was left out.

Today, thanks to lessons learned from mothers like Jacqueline Kennedy, the body of a baby like Patrick, who is transferred from the hospital of birth to another hospital for newborn intensive care and dies there, is often returned to the hospital of birth for his mother to see, to touch, and to hold. A funeral service can be held in the birth hospital chapel or postponed until the mother is discharged. In this way, both parents not only get the chance to say goodbye to their baby, but to say goodbye together.

One additional thought: Some people do not remember that three of Jacqueline Kennedy's five pregnancies ended in tragedy after she married John F. Kennedy in 1953:

- She suffered a miscarriage in 1955.
- A daughter, Arabella, was stillborn in 1956.
- Caroline was born full-term in 1957.
- John, Jr. was delivered four weeks early in 1960.
- Patrick was delivered five-and-a-half weeks early and lived for only 40 hours in 1963.

Jacqueline Kennedy gave birth to all of her children by cesarean section.

THE ALPHABET SOUP OF PREMATURE BABY CARE

Q *Our oldest daughter recently gave birth to our first grandchild. Normally, that would be cause for a celebration. The only problem is little Melissa was born premature (she weighed 3 pounds, 10 ounces) and was hooked up to a machine for two days to help her breathe. The doctors have reassured my daughter that Melissa will not have to go back on the machine and will likely be okay.*

D. Gary Benfield, M.D.

We talk by phone or by e-mail every day. During those conversations, my daughter uses so many abbreviations that it makes my head spin. When I ask her what such and such means, even she sometimes can't say for sure.

I could sure use your help with these three examples:

- *The doctors say Melissa is having As and Bs but not to worry because they are being controlled with medication. What are As and Bs?*
- *The doctors also say she has no evidence of IVH. What is IVH?*
- *Finally, they describe her breathing problem as RDS. Can you explain RDS in simple terms?*

A Welcome to the alphabet soup of premature baby care. If I can paraphrase, Melissa suffers from RDS, complicated by As and Bs, but, thankfully, she has no evidence of IVH.

RDS stands for *respiratory distress syndrome,* the most common breathing problem of premature babies. RDS is caused by insufficient surfactant, a substance produced by the lungs that spreads like a film, lining the millions of tiny air sacs and helping them stay open.

When a baby's lungs lack surfactant, the baby has to work harder than normal to breathe. In many cases, the baby soon tires out and stops breathing. That's why Melissa's doctors placed a breathing tube down her throat and attached the tube to a respirator to take over the work of breathing for her.

Most likely, her doctors also injected artificial surfactant down the breathing tube to help tide her over until her lungs started making adequate surfactant on their own. In Melissa's case, it took two days to happen, then she no longer needed respirator assistance.

A and B stand for *apnea* and *bradycardia.* Apnea is a pause in breathing that lasts for more than 15 to 20 seconds. Bradycardia is a slowing of the heart rate. Apnea and bradycardia occur commonly in premature babies. They are usually caused by immaturity of the breathing center in the brain.

As Melissa's brain matures, her tendency to have apnea and bradycardia will disappear. Most likely, it will happen before she is discharged from the hospital.

IVH stands for *intraventricular hemorrhage* or bleeding deep within the brain in the area where our spinal fluid is produced. Since the doctors have said Melissa doesn't have IVH, this means they have done an ultrasound of her brain and found it to be normal, a very good sign.

FACING THE CHALLENGE OF PREMATURE BIRTH

Q *My two-week-old daughter has been in a newborn intensive care unit since birth. She was born nine weeks early and spent the first three days on a breathing machine. The doctors and nurses all say she is doing fine, but having her there is making me crazy.*

Each time I visit, I start crying and thinking it's all my fault. Then I get to thinking they're not telling me everything. I can't imagine how I'm going to take care of her after she goes home. Can you please help me sort out these scary feelings?

A Take a deep breath and try to relax. Based on the information you've provided, your daughter was apparently born at 31 weeks gestation. (Full term is 40 weeks, and you said she was 9 weeks early.) Since she is now two weeks old, her "corrected" gestational age is 31 weeks plus 2 weeks, or 33 weeks. In other words, she is still 7 weeks early.

Most babies who are born this early and need help with their breathing for a couple of days are usually ready to go home around 35 or 36 weeks corrected gestational age. This means your daughter will probably be ready for discharge in two to three weeks.

Before we discuss the specific things you will need to do to get ready to take your daughter home, let's first discuss your feelings.

Studies show that most mothers who give birth to a premature baby believe it's their fault. Oftentimes, their "guilt trip" is reinforced by something they saw on television or the Internet or by free advice they received from family members or friends. Yet, in most cases, their baby's premature birth was simply beyond their control. It helps to look ahead and not dwell on the past.

You also question whether the doctors and nurses are telling you the truth about your daughter's condition. This concern is also common. Chances are the staff is being honest and sharing what they know.

Nowadays, nurses and doctors who care for premature newborns view parents as partners and don't withhold information from them about their babies. You might ask to speak with your baby's doctor and share your concerns.

Now, what goals must you and your baby accomplish for the two of you to go home together in several weeks?

- Your daughter must be able to coordinate her sucking, swallowing, and breathing while taking all her feedings by mouth before she can be weaned from her incubator to a crib.
- Once she has been weaned from the incubator to a crib, she will need to maintain her body temperature and stay free of any low heart rates (bradycardia) or periods of forgetting to breathe (apnea).
- Nowadays, there's no magic weight for her to reach before she can go home.

You might sit down with your daughter's nurse and, together, draw up a pre-discharge plan. The plan will include at least the following:

- Learning how to breastfeed or bottle feed your baby
- Learning how to take your daughter's temperature

- Learning how to change her diaper
- Learning how to give her a bath
- Learning how to use a car seat

Your daughter's nurse will also help you choose your daughter's follow-up doctor and help you make an appointment for her first well-baby checkup. This list may seem like a lot to accomplish in several weeks, but you can do it if you just tackle the plan one task at a time.

When discharge day rolls around, you will feel a great sense of accomplishment! But don't be surprised if you still feel a bit anxious and question your ability to care for your daughter at home. This reaction is normal and one that almost all parents of preemies go through at discharge. It too shall pass.

MASSAGE THERAPY HELPS PREEMIES GROW

Q *I read that massage therapy helps premature babies grow faster and go home from the hospital sooner than premature babies who are not massaged. Is this true? If so, can you explain why?*

A Dr. Tiffany Field did the pioneering work in this area. In one study, she showed that massaged and exercised preterm infants gained 47 percent more in weight than a preterm control group that was not massaged or exercised, even though both groups got the same number of feedings each day and averaged the same intake of formula. Also, the hospital stays of babies in the treated group were six days shorter than babies in the control group, saving about $3,000 on each treated baby's hospital bill.

We don't know precisely how massage helps preemies grow faster. Some researchers believe massage may improve the intestine's ability to absorb milk and convert it into the building blocks for growth.

D. Gary Benfield, M.D.

"KANGAROO CARE" HELPS PARENTS, PREEMIES BOND

Q *I recently read about kangaroo care, a new way for parents to bond with their premature babies. Can you explain the benefits of kangaroo care and how it got started?*

A Back in the 1970s, parents of premature newborns reluctantly sat on the sidelines and watched while specialized nurses assumed the parenting role. Today, the rules have changed. Thanks to skin-to-skin holding, nicknamed *kangaroo care,* parents are holding the tiniest babies and sharing in their care.

Kangaroo care started in the early 1980s in an overcrowded nursery in Bogota, Colombia. Faced with a shortage of incubators and an increasing number of deaths, doctors encouraged Colombian mothers to tuck their premature babies inside their blouses, skin-to-skin between their breasts, for hours at a time.

This skin-to-skin approach worked better than expected:

- The number of deaths dropped off.
- Kangaroo-care infants had shorter hospital stays.
- Fewer parents abandoned their babies.

These findings were later duplicated in Kenya and Mozambique.

Kangaroo care then found its way to the more developed nurseries of Europe. There, researchers confirmed those earlier findings and added some of their own:

- Kangaroo-care mothers were more likely to breastfeed their babies.
- They also grew more attached to their babies.
- They were more confident mothers after discharge.
- Kangaroo-care preemies grew faster and had shorter hospital stays.

Walking the Baby Beat

Kangaroo care is rapidly catching on in nurseries across the United States, so far with positive results. Dressed in a diaper, a hat, and a light blanket, and warmed by their parents' skin, stable infants as small as two pounds can be safely held by parents.

Recently, inside the neonatal intensive care unit at Akron Children's Hospital, a shirtless father was busy scrubbing his chest. "My wife and I take turns holding her skin-to-skin," he said. "After all, she's my daughter too."

A further thought: Famous movie star, Humphrey Bogart, was best known for playing tough guys. His father was a prominent New York surgeon, and his mother, Maud Humphrey, was a successful commercial artist who painted portraits of children. Baby Humphrey was said to have been her model when she painted the Gerber baby.

TREATING JAUNDICE OF PREMATURITY WITH FLUORESCENT LIGHT

Q *Almost five weeks ago, my wife blessed us with a beautiful baby girl. We named her Lindsay. She was born four weeks early and had to stay in the hospital for nine days before she was strong enough to come home.*

The only problem was she turned a deep yellowish-orange, what the doctor called "jaundice of prematurity." He was able to lower the jaundice level by putting her under a bank of fluorescent lights—with only a diaper on for clothing—for several days. After that, the remaining jaundice faded away. Now that she's home, she's doing fine.

I'm curious. Can you tell me who discovered that fluorescent light will lower a baby's jaundice level? Can you explain how these lights work in cases of jaundice? Regarding Lindsay, should we watch for any side effects?

A What you've just described is called *phototherapy*. The fascinating story of how phototherapy was discovered goes

D. Gary Benfield, M.D.

back to 1956 when Sister Ward, the nurse in charge of the premature baby unit at Rochford General Hospital in Essex, England, routinely took the more "delicate infants" out into the nearby courtyard. She thought the combination of fresh air and sunshine would do them more good than the stuffy, overheated atmosphere of their incubators.

One day she noticed a jaundiced, premature infant was also yellowish-orange, like your Lindsay, except for a triangular area of skin that was more yellow than the rest of her body. A corner of the sheet had covered this area, and Sister Ward concluded that the rest of the infant had been "bleached" by the sun.

A short time later, someone accidentally left a tube of a baby's blood exposed to sunlight for several hours. When the pigment that causes jaundice—known as bilirubin—was measured, it was much lower than before.

Sister Ward and her doctors then put two and two together and realized that visible light could lower serum bilirubin. Thus, the idea of using fluorescent light as a clinical tool to treat jaundice was born.

How does phototherapy work? When an infant is placed under a phototherapy light (the bank of fluorescent lights you described) or on a special light blanket, she receives a continuous dose of photons of energy. These photons are absorbed by bilirubin molecules in the skin, resulting in a chemical reaction that breaks down the bilirubin into smaller components. These breakdown products are excreted in the stool, which lowers the level of jaundice in the baby.

What about side effects? Phototherapy is remarkably safe. At this point, your daughter's jaundice has disappeared and won't return. There are no delayed side effects to watch for.

A further thought: Jaundiced, full-term infants have been safely treated with phototherapy at home for many years.

Home phototherapy avoids separating mother and baby, and is certainly cheaper than using it in the hospital. Of course, only healthy babies who no longer require hospital care qualify.

HOW DO YOU TELL WHETHER A BABY IS PREMATURE OR FULL TERM?

Q *How can you tell whether a newborn baby is full term or premature?*

A Before answering your question, let's first review the concept of gestational age, then define prematurity. A baby's gestational age is commonly assessed by one of three methods:

- Clinical dating
- Ultrasound measurements
- The newborn gestational age assessment

And, I might add, these three methods don't always agree. Confused already? Let me explain.

When a pregnant woman has her first prenatal visit, one of the first things her doctor asks is, "What was the first day of your last menstrual period?"

Armed with this date, the doctor can then figure out her due date. This method of determining gestational age is called clinical dating.

Now, the typical pregnancy, measured from the first day of the last menstrual period, lasts 280 days (40 weeks), plus or minus 14 days. So the doctor then takes out his calendar, counts forward 40 weeks from the first day of his patient's last menstrual period, and assigns that date as her due date.

But remember, the due date is 40 weeks, plus or minus 14 days or two weeks. So a full-term baby is defined as any baby born between 38 and 42 weeks gestation, with an average of 40 weeks. A baby born at 37 weeks gestation or less is defined as premature. Incidentally, a baby born later than 42 weeks gestation is called postmature.

If you notice, I have not mentioned the baby's birthweight. A baby can weigh 4 pounds and still be full-term while a baby can weigh 9 pounds and still be premature. The 4 pound, term baby is called *small for gestational age* while the 9 pound, premature baby is called *large for gestational age.*

To apply what we've learned about clinical dating, let's say you're pregnant, and the first day of your last menstrual period was January 16, 2006. If you count forward 40 weeks from January 16, your due date turns out to be October 23.

Ultrasound is also an accurate means of estimating gestational age, at least in the first half of pregnancy; measurements of fetal length, head size, and femur length correlate closely with gestational age. However, sometimes the gestational age obtained from clinical dating and ultrasound measurements disagree.

The final arbitrator, especially when the date of the mother's last menstrual period is uncertain, then becomes the gestational age assessment performed after the baby is born.

The gestational age of most newborns—based on the baby's neuromuscular and physical maturity—is assessed after birth using a scoring system developed by Dr. Jean Ballard, a neonatologist in Cincinnati. Here's how it works: A score of 40 points equates to 40 weeks gestation, 35 points to 38 weeks gestation, 30 points to 36 weeks gestation, 25 points to 34 weeks and so on. Obviously then, a baby must score 35 points or more to be considered full-term.

A further thought: Here's a friendly warning: Parents and doctors sometimes assume that a baby born at 37, 36, or even 35 weeks gestation can be treated like a full-term baby even though the baby is really premature. This error in judgment can lead to the following problems:

- Spitting up, from being fed too much or too often for the baby's age.
- Inability to maintain body temperature (hypothermia), from not being dressed warmly enough or being exposed to the cold when bathing, assuming the baby can handle it.
- Periods of prolonged pauses in breathing (apnea), from overfeeding and cold exposure, again assuming the baby is more mature than she actually is.
- Then the baby gets labeled as being "sick" and may undergo expensive tests and treatments and winds up staying longer in the hospital when, in fact, the baby is only acting like a normal premature baby.

Your newborn by the numbers

HOW'S YOUR NEWBORN IQ?

Let's have some fun with the following quiz. Circle your best guess. The answers are given at the end.

1. Approximately how many babies born in the United States are delivered by Cesarean section?
   a. 5%
   b. 15%
   c. 25%
   d. 30%

2. Almost 50 percent of newborns in the United States are breastfed at birth. How many are breastfed at six months?
   a. 40%
   b. 30%

c. 20%
d. 10%

3. The healthy adult takes 16 to 18 breaths each minute. How many breaths does the healthy newborn take per minute?
   a. 20
   b. 30
   c. 40
   d. 50

4. The healthy adult's heart beats 60–80 times each minute. How many times does the healthy newborn's heart beat per minute?
   a. 80–100
   b. 100–120
   c. 120–140
   d. 140–160

5. Some infants have a regular fussy period each day, particularly in the evening. When these episodes intensify and persist throughout the day, they are called *colic*. **How many babies develop colic?**
   a. 5%
   b. 10%
   c. 20%
   d. 30%

6. If you show your infant four identical toys, each of a different color, which toy will he look at the longest?
   a. blue
   b. yellow

c. red
d. green

7. By what age should your baby be able to hold up her head and chest as she supports herself on her elbows?
   a. Two months
   b. Three months
   c. Four months
   d. Five months

Answers: "c" is the answer to all seven questions. Seven correct answers is exceptional. Six is above average. Four or five is average. Less than four is below-average.

YOUR NEWBORN BY THE NUMBERS

- **140** The number of times your baby's heart beats each minute.
- **201,600** The number of times your baby's heart beats each day.
- **73,584,000** The number of times your baby's heart beats during the first year of life. In comparison, your heart beats about 70 times each minute, 100,800 times each day and 36,792,000 each year, about half the number of times your baby's heart beats during the first year of life.
- **40** The number of breaths your baby takes each minute.
- **57,600** The number of breaths your baby takes each day.
- **21,024,000** The number of breaths your baby will take during the first year of life.

D. Gary Benfield, M.D.

- **60** The average life expectancy in years for a baby born with Down syndrome.
- **18** The average number of hours a healthy newborn sleeps each day. By 12 months of age, a typical infant sleeps about 14 hours each day.
- **6** The average age in months when a baby's first tooth erupts.
- **1 in 87** The natural incidence of twin births in the United States.
- **9.9%, 11.2%, and 17.6%** The prematurity rates, in percent of births, for white, Hispanic, and black women, respectively, in this country.

Circumcision

SHOULD WE HAVE OUR BABY CIRCUMCISED?

Q *I am due in six weeks to have a baby boy. After he's born, my husband wants him circumcised, but I'm not so sure. My obstetrician, who would normally do the circumcision, says he will do whatever we want. Can you offer any guidance?*

A The difference of opinion between you and your husband sounds a bit like a the debate that has been going on nationally. It all started several years ago when the American Academy of Pediatrics (AAP) released a new policy statement on newborn circumcision. In essence, the AAP said the following:

- Existing scientific evidence suggests that newborn circumcision is beneficial, but the evidence isn't strong enough to recommend that all male newborns should be circumcised.

- Parents should decide what is in the best interest of their children.
- Parents should be given unbiased information and the opportunity to discuss the information in order to make an informed decision.
- If a decision for circumcision is made, the baby should receive adequate medication for pain.

At the time, the AAP's stance seemed reasonable enough to me, but, apparently, it wasn't reasonable to everyone. Some members of the mainstream media became convinced that the AAP had adopted an anticircumcision stance and took the AAP to task. But not all members of the media interpreted the new policy statement as a recommendation against circumcision, noting that the AAP had never advocated routine circumcision of newborns.

Here's my view on this controversial issue:

- **Newborn circumcision has several benefits:** It prevents urinary tract infection (UTI), penile cancer, constriction of the foreskin so it can't be pulled back, local infection, and sexually transmitted diseases, HIV in particular.
- **It also has several disadvantages:** potential pain of the procedure, cost, occasional postoperative bleeding and infection, and, rarely, a doctor has been known to make a mistake and cut off the tip of the penis.
- In an important, more recent study, researchers found that newborn circumcision lowered the incidence of UTI during the first year of life by ninefold when compared to uncircumcised infants. In addition, circumcised infants had markedly lower UTI-related medical costs and rate of hospital admissions.

In my opinion, this new information tilts the debate toward favoring circumcision, provided the doctor doing it can provide adequate pain relief.

A further thought: The American Academy of Pediatrics suggests that parents make their decision about circumcision with their doctor, preferably before birth. In that way, parents can avoid having to make a snap decision after their baby is born, under the pressure of early discharge.

HOW DO YOU TAKE CARE OF THE UNCIRCUMCISED PENIS?

Q *My wife and I have decided not to have our son circumcised after he is born. Can you explain daily care to keep his penis clean?*

A Before we discuss daily care of your son's penis, let me give you some background to help you understand what you will be doing.

Before birth, as the fetus grows, the tip of the penis or glans and the sleeve of skin that covers the glans, known as the foreskin, both develop as one tissue. That's why the foreskin is firmly attached to the glans at birth.

About the age of two, the foreskin begins to separate from the glans. As a result, cells are shed from beneath the foreskin and gradually work their way to the surface. This collection of cells is known as smegma.

The glans and foreskin usually become fully separated by the age of three. After that, it will be easy to pull back the foreskin.

It's normal then, not to be able to pull back the foreskin during the first few years of life, before separation is complete. If you forcefully try to pull back the foreskin before separation is complete, it will cause pain, bleeding, and swelling.

With this background in mind, care of the uncircumcised penis is easy. Good hygiene simply requires washing the penis with soap and water at bath time. The foreskin should be left alone and the smegma washed away.

When your son is older and separation is complete, you can teach him how to pull back his foreskin and wash his penis himself.

Twins and higher multiples

THE CASE OF THE VANISHING TWIN

Q *My sister recently gave birth to a beautiful baby girl, but earlier in her pregnancy, the doctor had said she was carrying twins. Can you tell me what happened to the other twin? Did the doctor make a mistake?*

A I doubt that anyone made a mistake. It may surprise you to know that early fetal ultrasound exams usually detect twins in about 4 of every 100 pregnancies. Yet, typically, twins are born just once in every 87 births. To rephrase your question, "What happens to the other twins?"

This phenomenon, known as the vanishing twin syndrome, occurs when one twin dies early in pregnancy and the surviving twin is later delivered as a single birth. Parents and doctors may be none-the-wiser unless an early ultrasound detects twins or careful examination of the placenta reveals fetal remains.

A further thought: Studies of twins support the importance of genes in the development of mood disorders. For instance, if one identical twin is diagnosed with a bipolar disorder the chance of the second twin developing the same problem is 67 percent. For nonidentical twins, the chances of the second twin developing the same problem drops to 20 percent, which is still much higher than the general population.

RAISING IDENTICAL TWINS

Q *Six months ago, my wife gave birth to identical twin boys. Ever since then, we have been bombarded with questions like "Why don't you put them in separate beds?" and "Why don't you dress them alike more often?"*

Feeling a bit overwhelmed, we could use your help with several issues: Will it cause any harm to let the boys share the same bed? Is it okay to dress them alike? Is it okay for them to be in the same class in school? Should they go off to the same college and room together?

A Hold on, let's not look too far ahead! By the time they are ready for college, your twin boys may have settled that issue themselves.

From experience, parents of identical twins strongly advise using the same principles to raise your sons as you would if they were born several years apart. Show each child an equal amount of love, kindness, and consideration. Be sensitive to each child's individual feelings. Accept and appreciate each one's distinctive behaviors. Praise and punish them individually.

If you want the boys to learn to sleep independently, put them in separate cribs before they begin to need each other to get to sleep at bedtime.

Even though infants do not care if they are dressed alike or differently, new parents of twins receive many duplicate sets of clothing as gifts. Most parents of identical twins are so proud of their babies, they enjoy dressing the babies alike in the early years. This also draws attention to the parents and makes them feel special.

Nearly all experienced parents of twins feel that dressing alike should stop when the boys reach school age. The right time is when they take an interest in choosing their own clothes. The important point is not how the boys are clothed but how they are treated. Dressing them alike makes it obvious to others that they are treated primarily as twins rather than individuals.

Schooling can be one of the big problems that parents of twins face. Teachers often prefer to separate twins because it is easier for them than trying to tell them apart and comparing their work. Based on the assumption that separation will promote individuality and independence, some schools have strict policies that require the separation of twins.

Yet, research seems to support routine placement together. Many parents of twins feel that separation should be the exception, not the rule, and that parents' opinions and their twins' desires should be respected. Shortly before your boys reach school age, plan ahead and meet with your school's principal after asking the boys what they prefer.

A further thought: Twins sometimes complain that Christmas and birthdays are not especially exciting because they tend to receive identical gifts. If Sam opens a package from Uncle John and finds a baseball glove, Ralph, who is watching, has a pretty good idea of what his present will be. Similarly, twins prefer to give separate gifts rather than giving one gift from the two of them.

DELIVERED, BUT STILL PREGNANT

Q *I recently heard of premature twins who were born weeks apart and survived. Is that true? If so, can you explain how it's possible?*

A Yes, it's true. But, for a good outcome, it takes the right set of circumstances and lots of luck.

Take, for example, Jennifer and Michael. They are indeed twins, but they don't share the same birthday. In fact, they weren't even born in the same year. Michael was born on December 12, 1995, and his twin sister Jennifer followed 91 days later on March 13, 1996.

When Susan, the twins' mother, went into labor at 26 weeks, her doctors tried everything possible to stop her labor. But when her water broke, Michael was born, weighing 2 pounds. At the time, his sister's estimated weight was 17 ounces and her chance for survival was very low.

Thanks to the drugs that had been used to try and stop the labor, or to Mother Nature, Susan's labor stopped before Jennifer was born. Because Jennifer's sac was still intact, the doctors sewed her mother's cervix shut and waited, hoping to gain even a few more days, perhaps a week or two. What they got was a miracle: three more months!

While Michael struggled to stay alive in the neonatal intensive care unit, his mother was confined to her hospital bed in another wing of the hospital. One month later, she was doing so well she was able to go home. "It was a strange feeling visiting Michael," she said. "Jennifer would be kicking inside me while Michael gripped my finger through a window in his incubator."

When Jennifer was born weighing 4 pounds, 15 ounces, Michael was still in intensive care, but doing much better. Though born 91 days apart, they went home from the hospital together.

ALL TWINS ARE NOT BORN EQUAL

Q *This is probably a dumb question, but can you tell me the difference between identical and fraternal twins? Are identical twins always the same sex?*

Walking the Baby Beat

A Basically, there are two types of twins: those born with identical genes (identical twins) and those born with different genes (fraternal twins). As a result, identical twins are always the same sex, whereas fraternal twins may be of the same or opposite sex.

A second difference is the way identical and fraternal twins are formed. Identical twins, just like a single baby, result from the union of one egg and one sperm at the moment of fertilization in the fallopian tube. Shortly after the fertilized egg, now a tiny mass of dividing cells called an embryo, enters the uterus, the embryo splits into two equal halves. Now two separate embryos, they implant in the wall of the uterus and grow as identical twins.

Before discussing how fraternal twins are formed, there's another rare type of identical twins—conjoined or Siamese twins. Conjoined twins result when the embryo fails to split completely, leaving the identical twins joined together, most commonly at the chest. Some conjoined twins live their lives joined together while others have been separated surgically.

Probably the most famous conjoined twins, Chang and Eng, were born connected at the chest in 1811 in Thailand, formerly known as Siam. Promoted as "Siamese Twins," they toured with Barnum's circus and became quite wealthy. In the late 1830s, they retired to North Carolina, married two sisters, Adelaide and Sarah Yates of Wilkes County, and ultimately fathered 21 children. Eng and Chang died two hours apart in January 1874, at the age of 63.

Fraternal twins are formed when two eggs, which may be from one or both ovaries, are fertilized by two different sperm. As you might expect, about 50 percent of fraternal twins are of mixed sex. In effect, this type of twinning results in a double birth, no different from siblings born years apart.

D. Gary Benfield, M.D.

Barbara and Jenna Bush, the daughters of Laura and George W. Bush, are fraternal twins. Born on November, 11, 1981, Barbara was born first, weighing 5 pounds, 4 ounces. Jenna weighed 4 pounds, 12 ounces.

Jenna underwent an emergency appendectomy on December 25, 2000, shortly before her father took office as president of the United States. As far as we know, Barbara still has her appendix. The twins graduated from college: Barbara from the University of Texas, Jenna from Yale University.

A further thought: In vitro fertilization has produced a virtual epidemic of twins and higher multiples, especially in this country. Fertility specialists commonly place anywhere from two to five budding embryos in a woman's uterus to increase the odds of a successful pregnancy. Most of the resulting offspring will be fraternal twins, fraternal triplets, and so on up the line. Occasionally, however, one of those budding embryos will split apart and result in identical twins or even triplets within the total number of offspring.

FUN FACTS ABOUT CELEBRITY TWINS

Twins have always aroused special interest, especially when they reach celebrity status. Conjoined or Siamese twins cause even more of a sensation. So let's explore the universe of twins and see what we can uncover.

Identical twins, Pauline Esther and Esther Pauline Friedman were born 17 minutes apart on July 4, 1918, in Des Moines, Iowa. At the age of 37, Esther started writing her Ann Landers advice column for the *Chicago Sun Times*. Not to be outdone by her "older" twin sister, Pauline decided she could write a column too. Three months later, she started writing her "Dear Abby" advice column for the *San Francisco Chronicle*.

Walking the Baby Beat

Early in their careers, the two columnists were often at odds, trying to top one another. Eventually, things got so bad they went for almost 10 years without talking to each other. However, they eventually got over their rift and grew closer before Ann Landers died of cancer in 2002.

In the world of sports, Jose and Ozzie Canseco both played Major League Baseball. Jose, the more successful of the two, played 17 seasons and hit 462 home runs. They were born in Havana, Cuba.

Harvey and Horace Grant both played basketball in the NBA. Horace had more success, playing for three championship teams with the Chicago Bulls and one with the Los Angeles Lakers.

Ashley and Mary-Kate Olsen are among the most famous and wealthy modern-day twins. The 19-year-old actors are currently pursuing their college degrees in New York. That's so cool.

Did you know that Mario Andretti, John Elway, and Alanis Morisette are twins? Similarly, Elvis Presley, Liberace, Ed Sullivan, Jim Thorpe, and Thornton Wilder were also twins. Elvis Presley's twin brother died at birth.

Let's not overlook famous women who have given birth to twins. They include Laura Bush, Margaret Thatcher, Madeline Albright, Ingrid Bergman, Loretta Lynn, Jane Seymour, Jane Pauley, Cybil Shepherd, Mia Farrow, and Cleopatra.

Famous fathers of twins include Nelson Rockefeller, Nat King Cole, Joseph Kennedy, Roy Rogers, Jimmy Stewart, Andy Williams, George Bush, Steve Forbes, Mel Gibson, James Taylor, Ray Romano, Michael Douglas, Muhammad Ali, Robert DeNiro, Al Pacino, Ed Asner, Bing Crosby, Andy Williams, Michael J. Fox, Lee Majors, Donald Sutherland, Denzel Washington, Malcolm X, and William Shakespeare.

Chang and Eng, the original "Siamese" twins, were born in 1811 in Siam, which later became Thailand after World War II. Joined at their upper abdomens, they acquired two managers as teens and performed for eager audiences around the world.

In England, for instance, they entertained royalty by playing shuttlecock, hitting a small cork ball with feathers back and forth. Audiences oohed and aahed as Chang and Eng moved across the floor with the ease and grace of a couple skillfully waltzing. They also answered questions in fluent English.

While still in their mid-20s, they retired to Wilkesboro, North Carolina, where they operated a general store. In 1839, Chang and Eng became American citizens and acquired their new name of Bunker.

About this time, they started dating the Yates sisters, Sallie and Adelaide. After several years, the foursome was married, moved into a new house, and shared a large bed built for four.

In all, Eng and Sallie had 11 children, while Chang and Adelaide had 10. However, as their families grew larger and times grew harder, they ran into problems.

The two sisters fought, putting Eng and Chang in the middle. Soon, the brothers turned against each other and more fights erupted. That's when they decided they needed separate homes.

They built their homes less than a mile apart and started a new routine. The wives and their respective children lived apart while Chang and Eng rotated, three days at a time, living at each other's home. This arrangement continued for the rest of their lives.

In order to support their families, Chang and Eng went on tour for up to a year at a time, each taking a child who also performed in their show.

Finally, on January 17, 1874, Eng woke up to find his brother cold. When he realized Chang was dead, Eng became ill and died a few hours later.

Today, the relatively minor surgical procedure required to separate them could be done easily by a general surgeon.

Genetics and birth defects

CAN TWO BROWN-EYED PARENTS HAVE A CHILD WITH BLUE EYES?

Q *Our biology teacher said two brown-eyed parents can have a child with blue eyes, but I don't understand how it works. Can you explain how this works?*

A It works only if both brown-eyed parents carry the recessive gene for blue eyes. Here's what I mean.

The genes for traits such as eye color occur in pairs on our chromosomes. Let's say B is the gene for brown eyes and b is the gene for blue eyes. If a person's gene-pair for eye color is BB, she will have brown eyes. If her gene-pair for eye color is bb, she will have blue eyes. But if her gene-pair for eye color is Bb, she will have brown eyes because B dominates b. Put another way, b is recessive to B.

If a brown-eyed male's sperm carrying the BB gene-pair for eye color fertilizes a brown-eyed female's egg carrying the BB gene-pair for eye color, four combinations are possible: each one is BB. And all their children will have brown eyes.

On the other hand, if one brown-eyed parent's gene-pair for eye color is Bb and the other parent's is BB, the four possible combinations are BB, Bb, BB, and Bb. Again, each of their children will have brown eyes because B dominates b.

But if both brown-eyed parents carry the gene-pair Bb, the four possible combinations are BB, Bb, Bb and bb. In this case, each of their children will have a 1-in-4 chance of inheriting the gene-pair bb, which causes blue eyes. Your biology teacher was probably talking about this special case.

A further thought: Brown eyes, farsightedness, and dimples dominate blue eyes, nearsightedness, and freckles in the world of dominant-recessive genes.

D. Gary Benfield, M.D.

WHAT HAPPENS TO THE REMOVED FLUID AFTER AN AMNIOCENTESIS?

Q *When a doctor does an amniocentesis and takes fluid from around the baby, what does the doctor do with the fluid to tell whether the baby has some kind of genetic problem?*

A The fetus constantly sheds skin cells into the amniotic fluid. When a sample of amniotic fluid is placed in a test tube and spun at a high rate of speed in a centrifuge, a small button of fetal skin cells forms at the bottom. These skin cells are then processed in the laboratory, yielding a karyotype or blown-up picture of a cell's chromosomes. By studying this picture, a geneticist can tell whether the baby has an extra chromosome. Down syndrome, for instance, is caused by an extra chromosome #21.

These skin cells can also be tested for a mutation in one of the thousands of genes that reside on the chromosomes. The gene mutation for cystic fibrosis, for example, can be detected in this way.

A further thought: The human body contains approximately 100 trillion (million million) cells, most of which are less than a tenth of a millimeter across. Inside each cell is a central blob called a nucleus. Inside the nucleus are a pair of 23 chromosomes, in total 46, which contain two complete sets of the human genome (except in egg cells and sperm cells, which have one copy each, and red blood cells, which have none). One set of the genome came from the mother and one from the father.

Imagine the genome is a book. In the book are 23 chapters, called chromosomes. Each chapter contains several thousand stories called genes. Each word is written in letters called bases. The 1 billion words in the book make it as long as 800 bibles. Two of these gigantic documents fit inside the microscopic nucleus of a tiny cell that fits easily upon the head of a pin.

WHAT ARE MY BABY'S CHANCES OF HAVING DOWN SYNDROME?

Q *I'm 36 years old and just found out I'm pregnant. Can you tell me what the chances are that my baby has Down syndrome?*

A Your risk of having a baby with Down syndrome increases with age, as shown in the following statistics:

- At age 25, the risk is 1 in 1,300 births.
- At age 30, it is 1 in 965 births.
- At age 35, it is 1 in 365 births.
- At age 40, it is 1 in 109 births.
- At age 45, it is 1 in 32 births.

Just to show another way to answer your question, the chances that a 35-year-old woman *will not* have a baby with Down syndrome are 364 out of 365 births, or 99.7 percent. Even at age 40, 108 out of 109 births or 99.1 percent *will not* have Down syndrome. You should ask your doctor for more details at your next checkup.

CAN YOU EXPLAIN THE FRAGILE X SYNDROME?

Q *Recently, a volunteer came through our neighborhood soliciting donations for research on the fragile X syndrome. Can you explain what it is?*

A Having a child with the fragile X syndrome can be a parent's worst nightmare. Imagine this fairly typical scenario:

D. Gary Benfield, M.D.

Your pregnancy couldn't have gone more smoothly. Your baby seems normal and healthy at birth. He smiles, coos, and sits at the right times. But as he passes his first birthday, you sense something is wrong.

When you try to read a story to him, he jumps down from your lap and runs away. He develops the habit of chewing his hands, has difficulty making eye-to-eye contact, and, no matter how hard you try, he just won't listen or follow the simplest instructions. His speech may be delayed. And when he does learn to talk, he repeats, repeats, repeats.

You may wonder: Am I a bad parent or is he a bad child? When you take your concerns to your doctor, she may pass them off as typical boy kinds of behavior. Or, if she takes them seriously, she may overlook the possibility that your son has fragile X. Increasingly frustrated, you may go from doctor to doctor before one finally orders a blood test and makes the diagnosis.

The fragile X syndrome is the most common cause of inherited mental retardation. It affects 1 in 2,000 males, while 1 in 259 women are carriers. Typically, fragile X children have developmental delays, autistic behavior, are hyperactive, and have a shortened attention span. Many are diagnosed with attention deficit disorder and placed on medication.

Only 50 percent of fragile X patients show the telltale physical characteristics that can help make the diagnosis easier. These features include large, prominent ears; an elongated face; hyperextensible joints; enlarged testicles; and flat feet.

The fragile X syndrome is caused by a mutation—a change in the DNA structure of a gene—at a fragile site on the X chromosome. As you may know, every cell in our bodies, except red blood cells, contains 46 chromosomes. Two are sex chromosomes: XX for girls, XY for boys.

Seventy percent of girls who carry the fragile X mutation on one of their X chromosomes show no signs of the disorder, because their other normal X chromosome balances out any ill effects. However, up to 30 percent of these carriers may be mildly affected. Having only one X chromosome, affected boys all show signs of the full-blown disorder.

Experts predict that in 10 to 15 years a genetically engineered replacement therapy for the fragile X gene will be available. Meanwhile, early diagnosis and early intervention, as well as genetic counseling for parents, remain the mainstays of treatment for children with fragile X.

A further thought: Mary Higgins Clark, known as the "Queen of Suspense" for her best-selling mystery novels, is the grandmother of a teenager with fragile X syndrome. She pledged $1 million to support further research.

WHEN COUSINS PLAN TO MARRY

Q *My cousin and I are third-year college students and have been dating seriously for about a year. We plan to get married right after graduation. Can you tell us what the risk of birth defects might be for our children? Also, do you know whether cousin marriages are legal in Ohio?*

A In general, the risk of noncousin couples having a child with a genetic disorder is 3–4 percent. For cousin couples, the risk increases slightly by an additional 1–2 percent. Each couple's situation, cousins or not, is unique, depending on the family medical history.

The two of you should seriously consider consulting a genetic counselor. She will ask questions about your family medical history; draw up a pedigree (like a family tree), going back several generations; and estimate your risk of having a child with a serious genetic problem.

The legal status of cousin marriages in the United States varies from state to state. Nineteen states allow cousin marriages; nineteen states prohibit them; and twelve states prohibit them with certain exceptions, according to Cousincouples.com.

The state of Ohio falls in the last category. To be on the safe side, if you plan to marry in Ohio, consult an attorney.

A further thought: Some state laws that prohibit cousin marriages are really bizarre. For instance, a few states that prohibit cousin marriages will recognize your marriage in another state. So far, so good. But other states that prohibit cousin marriages will not recognize your marriage in another state. It is very important to find out what your home state's policy is if you plan on marrying in another state. Why? Your home state might accuse you of attempting to evade the laws of your state. If convicted, you can be fined and possibly serve jail time.

THE RISK OF HAVING A SECOND BABY WITH CYSTIC FIBROSIS

Q *Our first child was born with cystic fibrosis. My home pregnancy test turned positive this morning, so I guess I'm pregnant again. Can you tell me what my chances are of having another baby with cystic fibrosis?*

A Your chances are as follows:

- 1 in 4 of having a baby with cystic fibrosis.
- 2 in 4 of your baby being a carrier of cystic fibrosis.
- 1 in 4 that your baby will not be a carrier or have the disease.

You should make an appointment to see your doctor as soon as possible to confirm the pregnancy test result. If it's positive, you and your doctor have a few things to discuss, including your need for genetic counseling.

A further thought: I was recently asked whether taking anticonvulsant drugs during pregnancy increases the risk of cleft lip and cleft palate in the baby.

Substantial evidence shows that anticonvulsant drugs, such as Dilantin, increase by two- to threefold the incidence of cleft lip and cleft palate when compared with the general population.

This statistic points out the importance of pre-pregnancy counseling before a woman becomes pregnant. Pre-pregnancy counseling allows the healthcare provider time to review any health problems and time to help a woman develop a plan for managing these problems to ensure the best outcome for mother and baby. Waiting until a woman discovers she is pregnant may be too late.

WHAT IS THE LIFE EXPECTANCY OF CHILDREN WITH DOWN SYNDROME?

Q *My nephew is almost two years old and has Down syndrome. Can you tell me how long children with Down syndrome can expect to live, and what they eventually die from?*

A The average life expectancy of a child born with Down syndrome now exceeds 60 years, according to Aubrey Milunsky, M.D., Director of the Center for Human Genetics at Boston University School of Medicine. This relatively long life expectancy means that brothers and sisters or other family members usually wind up caring for children with Down syndrome in old age. If no family members are willing or able to take on this responsibility, the state usually ends up as guardian.

Adults with Down syndrome tend to age prematurely and are more likely to develop early Alzheimer's disease than the general population. Complications such as leukemia (20 times more common in persons with Down syndrome, compared to the general population), diabetes, and serious infections often claim their lives. Adults with Down syndrome are also more likely to develop hearing loss, cataracts, glaucoma, and thyroid disorders.

A further thought: Now that more and more premature babies born weighing less than two pounds are surviving and going home, an increasing number of researchers are turning their attention to how well these babies do.

According to a study published in a recent issue of the *Journal of the American Medical Association*, neurologic damage in very small premature infants may actually decrease over time. Many youngsters once considered as doing poorly ended up scoring in the nearly normal range on tests of verbal function and IQ, the study found.

However, highly respected Cleveland researcher, Dr. Maureen Hack, is skeptical of these results. She worries that the children studied were not given tests designed to measure problems usually linked with extreme prematurity, such as attention deficits and visual-motor impairments.

These kinds of long-term follow-up studies are important but very difficult to do. They require hard work, lots of money, and parents who keep their appointments. This study shows promising results, but more studies are needed before we can draw any useful conclusions.

WHAT ARE MY BABY'S CHANCES OF INHERITING SICKLE CELL DISEASE?

Q *I'm African American and 12 weeks pregnant. Blood tests show that I carry the sickle cell trait. Can you tell me what the chances are of my baby inheriting sickle cell disease?*

A For a child to inherit sickle cell disease—a painful, disabling blood disorder that strikes 1 in 700 African Americans—both parents must carry the gene that causes it. This carrier state, known as sickle cell trait, affects 1 in 12 African Americans and is what you have.

Before your question can be fully answered, the father of your baby should be tested to see whether he carries the trait or has sickle cell disease. Chances are he doesn't have the disease because he would have symptoms, and you would have mentioned it.

Individuals who carry the sickle cell trait usually lead normal lives. If the father of your baby turns out to have sickle cell trait, your baby will have the following possible outcomes:

- 1-in-4 chance of inheriting sickle cell disease
- 2-in-4 chance of having sickle cell trait
- 1-in-4 chance of not having either one

On the other hand, if the father of your baby does not have sickle cell trait, then your baby has the following possible outcomes:

- 2-in-4 chance of having sickle cell trait
- 2-in-4 chance of being normal

So the worst-case scenario is your baby's father turns out to have sickle cell trait. Then your baby would have a 1-in-4 chance of having sickle cell disease and a 2-in-4 chance of sickle cell trait. Otherwise, if your baby's father doesn't have sickle cell trait, the worst thing that can happen is a 2-in-4 chance of your baby having sickle cell trait.

Once your baby's father receives his test results, the two of you should meet with your doctor to discuss their implications for your baby.

BREAKING BAD NEWS

The morning started off like most winter mornings in northeast Ohio. I started a pot of coffee, slipped on my coat and boots, and tip-toed down our ice-covered driveway to retrieve the morning paper. But, before I could savor my coffee or read the news, my beeper went off.

"Dr. Benfield, I'm taking care of a little girl who was born last night by cesarean section. My partner attended the delivery and examined the baby right after birth. She thought the baby had some features of Down syndrome but didn't say anything to the parents. She thought it was better to wait and see what I thought.

"The baby was born a few weeks early but is doing fine. She does have a few signs of Down syndrome. But like I told the parents, I'm not totally sure. Obviously, they're in a state of shock. They had no idea anything was wrong with their baby. If you wouldn't mind consulting, it would sure help us out."

I asked the caller a few questions then told him I could see the baby within the hour, if that was all right.

I arrived at the hospital as promised and headed for the nursery. The baby in question was out with her mother, so I decided to examine her in the mother's room. That way, her parents could watch what I was doing, I could point out my findings, and they could ask questions as I went along.

In the hallway outside the mother's room, I encountered a bright-eyed little boy and a woman who looked like she had been crying. She introduced herself as the baby's grandmother and the little boy as the baby's brother. I shook the little boy's hand and asked him how old he was. He held up three fingers and smiled. Then he said, "I holded her" and smiled again.

I knocked on the mother's door and went in. The blinds were closed and the lights were off inside the darkened room. Mom was propped up in bed. Intravenous fluids were running in one arm while she held her baby in the other. Her husband sat in a chair nearby. They were expecting me and seemed eager to know what I thought.

We turned on the lights and opened the blinds; I could tell they too had been crying. They seemed pleased that I

Walking the Baby Beat

was going to examine their baby there on mom's bed. Of course, before I could get started, dad and I had to change the baby's diaper.

I sat down and asked the couple what they understood so far.

Dad said their pediatrician was concerned their baby might have Down syndrome, but wasn't sure. Mom said she thought the baby looked just like her son after he was born. She also said she couldn't understand why something like this—if her baby did have Down syndrome—wasn't diagnosed before the baby was born.

I explained that even though most birth defects are diagnosed before birth, we still have a few surprises in the delivery room.

I started my exam at the top and worked down, talking to them as I went along. I pointed out how the back of her head was flat and how she kept flicking her tongue in and out. I mentioned these can be subtle signs of Down syndrome. I pointed out her flat nasal bridge, her up-slanted eyes, and the single crease across the palms of her hands. I mentioned these too may be signs of Down syndrome. I also said I didn't hear a heart murmur, an important negative finding since 25 percent or more of babies born with Down syndrome have some sort of congenital heart disease.

I finished my exam, bundled her up and handed her to her mother. Then I sat down and gathered my thoughts.

"Clinically, your baby has Down syndrome," I said, glancing from mom to dad. "We will need to do some blood tests to confirm the diagnosis."

Obviously disappointed, they did their best to hold back the tears. I answered a few questions then got up and headed for the door.

"The two of you need some private time," I said. "I'll come back after I've written a note in the chart and made a few phone calls."

I pulled the door shut behind me and paused for a moment. Their sobbing sent chills down my spine.

I wrote up my consult and told the nurses what I had said. Then I called mom's obstetrician and her baby's pediatrician to let them know I had confirmed their suspicions.

I returned to mom's room and resumed our conversation. Amazingly enough, mom and dad had dried their tears and seemed eager to deal with what came next. They had lots of questions about their daughter's future.

I explained she would probably roll over, sit up and walk later than her brother did. Mom asked, "Will she ever talk?" "Of course," I said. "It will just take longer than it did for your son to begin saying words."

We discussed the fact that she will be mentally retarded and need special schooling. I emphasized, however, that strong family support will be a key factor in helping her achieve her potential, just like it will be for their son to reach his potential.

I also pointed out she was acting no different than any other newborn. I suggested they try to treat her the same way they did their son when he was her age. "She's not fragile; she won't break," I said. They seemed to understand and also seemed relieved.

I helped them make an appointment with the Genetics Center at Akron Children's Hospital for counseling and to have the blood tests done. We also arranged for a heart specialist to see their baby the same day, just in case.

After answering more questions, we hugged and said our goodbyes.

Two hours had passed since I first arrived in the nursery. I had done the best I could. Now, it was up to them.

WHY IS MY HEART ON THE LEFT SIDE OF MY CHEST?

Q *One of the kids in school asked two questions in class that no one, including our teacher, could answer. Can you explain why the heart forms on the left side of the chest and not the* *right? Also, why is the liver on the right side of the abdomen and not the left?*

A The ultimate location of every organ in our body is determined by our genes. Your heart is located on the left side of your chest while your liver is located on the right of your abdomen because, early in pregnancy, the tissues that make up these organs were directed to form in those locations by controlling genes.

Mutations within these genes may result in a change of positioning—for example, in a right-sided heart and a left-sided liver. This rare disorder (called situs inversus) has been recognized as recessive, meaning when both parents have the mutation each offspring has a 1-in-4 chance of having situs inversus and a 3-in-4 chance of normal organ placement.

By the way, brain development favoring right-handedness and control of speech in the left side of the brain is probably also dictated by genes yet to be discovered.

A further thought: While we're on the subject of why things happen, have you ever noticed in pictures of the early embryo that the hands and feet develop as pads, with the fingers and toes firmly knitted together? How, one might ask, are those pads transformed into separate fingers and toes?

About the tenth week of pregnancy, when the growing embryo measures about 1 inch in length, the cells binding the fingers and toes together begin to die, allowing the digits to separate. This programmed cell death (called apoptosis) is controlled by specific genes. A mutation in a gene that controls this process may result in a child being born with one or more fingers or toes stuck together in a condition called syndactyly. Curiously, the second and third toes are the digits most frequently stuck together, or webbed.

Without programmed cell death, your heart would not have four hollow chambers, your intestine would not be a hollow tube, and your arteries and veins would not form as hollow channels to allow blood to flow through them. All of these events are under the control of genes. So programmed cell death is a part of life.

By the way, if you're a high school student wondering what to do for a career, there's no better place to start than to take a course in developmental biology. This fascinating subject pulls together embryology—the study of how animals develop during early life—and the science of genetics.

If you want to learn about the miracle of life: DNA and how genes function, or stem cells, cloning, inherited diseases, and so much more, it's all included in a course on developmental biology. Who knows, you might find yourself pursuing one of many careers that depend on knowing about this fascinating subject.

FOLIC ACID OR FOLATE: WHICH PREVENTS BIRTH DEFECTS BEST?

Q *I'm confused. Can you explain the difference between folate and folic acid, the vitamin pregnant women take to prevent birth defects? Does a vegetarian who eats lots of green vegetables have to take extra folic acid when she gets pregnant?*

A There are two main differences between folate and folic acid:

- First, folate is the naturally occurring form of a B-vitamin essential for growing cells. It is found in dark-green, leafy vegetables (spinach, collard greens, turnip greens, and romaine lettuce), broccoli, asparagus, beans, peanuts, strawberries, kiwi, and orange juice. On the other hand, folic acid is a manufactured or synthetic form of folate that is

now added to most breakfast cereals, bread, rice, pasta, and multivitamins.
- The second and most important difference, surprisingly enough, is that almost all of the folic acid we consume is absorbed in our intestine and available for our body's use. In contrast, less than 20 percent of the folate we consume is absorbed in our intestine and used by our body. So it's very difficult, even for a vegetarian, to consume enough folate daily to significantly reduce the risk of having a baby with a birth defect.

A further thought: While we're on the subject, it's important to remember that supplementing your diet with 0.4 mg of folic acid daily (the amount found in most multivitamin pills) *before you get pregnant* will reduce the risk by up to 70 percent of your unborn baby developing a neural tube defect.

So let's take a moment to understand what the neural tube is, what happens when it forms incorrectly, and why it's important to start taking 0.4 mg of folic acid daily *before you get pregnant.*

On or about the eighteenth day after conception, a tiny groove, called the neural groove, forms on the backside of the developing embryo, your unborn baby. At this point, your unborn baby is only about an eighth of an inch long.

Over the next 10 days, the neural groove pinches in at the middle and closes upward toward what will become your unborn baby's head and downward toward what will become your unborn baby's lower spinal column. (Think of a two-headed zipper that starts in the middle and closes at both ends.)

By the twenty-eighth day after conception, at a time when most women are unaware they're pregnant, the neural groove closes completely, forming the neural tube. At this point, your unborn baby is less than a quarter inch long.

D. Gary Benfield, M.D.

When all goes well, the top end of the closed neural tube develops into your unborn baby's brain and skull while the remainder of the neural tube becomes your baby's spinal column. However, in one out of 1,000 pregnancies, the neural tube fails to close completely, resulting in a neural tube defect.

When the neural tube fails to close at the head end, one of two possible neural tube defects results:

- One is called anencephaly, an always fatal problem. The skull fails to close, leaving a mass of nonfunctioning brain tissue showing through.
- The other possibility is called an encephalocele, an often fatal problem. Only part of the skull doesn't close, leaving a hole through which part of the brain protrudes, enclosed within a sac. Those babies who do survive often have severe physical and mental handicaps.

When the neural tube fails to close at the tail end, spina bifida or an open spine defect results. These babies need surgery soon after birth to close their open back and will often need a second surgery right away to drain their hydrocephalus or water on the brain.

These children usually face a lifetime of chronic health problems that require multiple surgeries. However, 80 to 90 percent of babies born with spina bifida survive, and many lead productive lives.

In summary:

- Folate is the naturally occurring form of an important B-vitamin, and folic acid is the synthetic form of folate.
- Folic acid is much better absorbed and used by the body than folate.
- All women of child-bearing age, even vegetarians, should supplement their diet *before getting pregnant*

with a daily multivitamin that contains 0.4 milligrams of folic acid to reduce their chances by up to 70 percent of giving birth to a baby with a neural tube defect.

NOT ALL BIRTH DEFECTS SHOW UP AT BIRTH

Q *Two weeks ago, my sister-in-law gave birth to a beautiful little girl. The doctor said she was fine. But several days later, she had trouble breathing and was put back in the hospital. Her new doctor discovered that her stomach had pushed through a hole in her diaphragm and was up in her chest, pressing on her lungs. I think he called it a diaphragmatic hernia. He said she needed an operation to fix it.*

She had the operation, and it was a success. She'll be going home in the next few days. Can you tell me why the first doctor didn't discover the problem at birth?

A Most babies born with a diaphragmatic hernia have difficulty breathing in the delivery room, making them relatively easy to diagnose. But they also have the worst prognosis. Why?

Because their intestines have been up in the chest, pressing on the baby's developing lungs, for weeks to months. As a result, their lungs are quite small and underdeveloped at birth. So even with emergency surgery, more than half of them will die.

The reason your niece's diaphragmatic hernia wasn't diagnosed sooner is because only a small portion of her intestines had recently slipped through the hole in her diaphragm, up into her chest, and hadn't been there long enough to seriously impair her developing lungs.

As a result, she didn't develop symptoms until after going home from the hospital. My guess is she has been given an excellent prognosis. Count your blessings.

D. Gary Benfield, M.D.

A further thought: A congenital anomaly—commonly called a birth defect—is a structural defect of an organ that is present at birth. It may be visible to the eye or hidden away within the body. Single minor anomalies are present in about 14 percent of newborns. These anomalies are of no serious medical consequence, but they alert the clinician to the possible presence of an associated major anomaly.

About 3 percent of all newborns have an obvious major anomaly at birth. Additional anomalies are detected later; thus the cumulative incidence is about 6 percent in two-year-olds and 8 percent in five-year-olds. Other anomalies (about 2 percent) are detected even later in life, during surgery or at autopsy.

WHY IS THIS TWO-DAY-OLD TURNING BLUE WITH FEEDING?

You are the doctor on duty in the emergency room when you get a frantic call from the nursery. A two-day-old baby has suddenly turned blue and gone limp in his mother's arms while feeding.

You rush to the nursery and administer oxygen and start an IV. The baby gradually pinks up, and his tone improves.

You must rule out a serious infection, so you draw some blood, do a spinal tap, and collect a urine specimen. Then you send the samples off to the lab and start antibiotics. Then you transfer the baby to the special care nursery for further evaluation and treatment.

You calm down the baby's mother and try to gather a clearer history. The baby was born two days ago and did well in the delivery room. The first six or eight bottle feedings were taken eagerly. But after that, the baby seemed a bit less interested in eating. Then, with this last feeding, the mother says her baby turned blue and became limp after taking about an ounce of formula.

Walking the Baby Beat

The baby has had normal bowel movements and six to eight wet diapers over the past 24 hours and no fever. Something doesn't add up here; it's sounding less and less like an infection.

In the special care nursery, the baby is sleeping comfortably. His physical exam is now completely normal. So far his lab tests show no signs of infection. His lungs are clear by X-ray, and his heart size is normal.

You ask yourself about other possibilities. Seizures in infants may take strange forms. Perhaps a subtle seizure caused the infant to go limp and change color. Gastric reflux is another possibility. After all, he did turn blue while feeding. You decide to see for yourself and feed the baby.

At first, he sucks eagerly. But after a few gulps, his color changes from pink to blue and his heart rate drops. You stop the feeding, give oxygen by mask, and stimulate him gently. He cries and turns pink.

No doubt, his problem is brought on by feeding. Because infants this age can only breathe through their nose, could a blocked nasal passage be causing his problem?

You easily pass a catheter down his right nostril. But when you try to pass the catheter down the left side, you meet resistance. With a little pressure you feel a pop and the catheter passes through. You have ruptured a congenital membrane; The medical term is *unilateral choanal atresia*. You have diagnosed and solved the baby's problem, all at the same time.

Babies born with unilateral choanal atresia may not have symptoms at birth: A problem develops later with feeding or when the open nasal passage is narrowed from a simple cold. However, the blockage is usually caused by a bony plate—requiring surgery—and not by a membrane. In this case, you were lucky; your attempt to pass the catheter not only made the diagnosis but also solved the problem.

Medical textbooks say this type of birth defect is rare, occurring once in every 5,000 births. But when you realize 4 million babies are born annually in the United States, it amounts to 800 babies born annually with choanal atresia, or more than two each day. When you put it this way, it doesn't seem rare at all.

Breastfeeding your baby

IS BREASTFEEDING SAFE WHEN MOM HAS THE FLU?

Q *I'm sick with the flu and breastfeeding my baby. My mother says I should stop nursing until I get well. I thought it was safe to breastfeed during an illness like this. Who is right?*

A Ordinarily, when nursing mothers develop a viral illness, it's safe to continue breastfeeding. There's always a chance that your baby will catch your illness, but passing on a virus can happen even if the baby weren't being nursed. Besides, viral infections are usually contagious well before symptoms develop. If you are coughing and sneezing, consider wearing a mask.

VACCINATING YOUR BREASTFEEDING INFANT

Q *I'm breastfeeding my baby, and he's due for his first immunizations. Is it okay for a breastfeeding baby to get his scheduled immunizations, or should they be postponed?*

A Breastfeeding is not a reason to postpone scheduled immunizations, for mother or for baby.

IS AMOXICILLIN SAFE FOR BREASTFEEDING MOTHERS?

Q *I'm breastfeeding my baby. My dentist prescribed amoxicillin before and after I have some dental work done. Can you* *tell me if amoxicillin will pass into my breast milk and possibly harm my baby?*

A Amoxicillin is excreted into breast milk in small amounts, but the American Academy of Pediatrics (AAP) considers amoxicillin safe for breastfeeding infants.

A further thought: The AAP warns that breastfeeding may be unsafe for mothers taking lithium. Lithium-induced toxicity in newborns can cause an irregular heart beat, heart enlargement, seizures, and shock.

DO BREAST IMPLANTS INTERFERE WITH BREASTFEEDING?

Q *I'm 24 and eventually plan to marry and have children. I am seriously thinking about having my breasts surgically enlarged. Can you tell me whether breast implants interfere with breastfeeding?*

A With modern surgical techniques, most women are able to successfully breastfeed after implant surgery. Here are some facts to help you understand what's involved and to increase your chances:

- Normally, two things are necessary for successful breastfeeding: an adequate number of milk ducts to supply the milk and a generous supply of nerves leading from the nipple and surrounding tissue. When the baby sucks, these nerves signal the brain to release hormones necessary for the let-down reflex and milk production.
- Any surgical procedure that cuts or damages these ducts or nerves will reduce the possibility of successful breastfeeding.
- Since there is more than one approach to implant surgery, make sure your surgeon understands how you feel about breastfeeding.

- Ask which approach involves the least damage to milk ducts and major nerves.
- Be sure to ask your questions before the surgery is done.

For those women who might be considering breast reduction surgery, the surgery often affects your ability to breastfeed because sections of the breast (including the milk ducts and major nerves) will be removed. Here again, there is more than one approach to breast reduction surgery.

Make your desires known about breastfeeding, and ask which approach will minimize damage to milk ducts and major nerves. Ultimately, the only way a mother who has undergone breast reduction surgery can find out whether her baby will receive enough milk through breastfeeding is to give it a try.

Finally, what if a mother needs a breast biopsy performed or a tumor or cyst removed? She too should talk to her surgeon about her desire to breastfeed. Ask the surgeon to avoid—within reason—cutting milk ducts and major nerves during the surgery.

THE LET-DOWN REFLEX

Q *When my baby sucks at one breast, milk dribbles out the other one. Can you explain why it happens?*

A When your baby sucks your breast, this action stimulates the nerve endings in the nipple to send messages to your brain. These messages stimulate the release of oxytocin from the pituitary gland. In turn, the oxytocin stimulates the muscle cells that surround the milk-producing cells in your breasts. When these muscle cells contract, milk is ejected from both nipples, not just the one your baby is sucking. This phenomenon is beyond your conscious control. It's called the let-down reflex.

IS PROPANALOL SAFE FOR BREASTFEEDING MOTHERS?

Q *I make my living playing the violin in a symphony orchestra and take a small dose of propanalol once or twice a week for performance anxiety. I'm also breastfeeding my baby. Can you tell me whether propanalol passes through into breast milk? Might it harm my baby?*

A Propanalol is excreted in small amounts in breast milk. However, based on studies of mothers taking much larger doses daily than you take in a week, propanalol is safe for mothers to take while breastfeeding, according to the American Academy of Pediatrics.

SHOULD WOMEN BREASTFEED IN PUBLIC?

Q *Would you please settle an argument between my mother-in-law and me? After my baby is born, I plan on breastfeeding, including the times when my husband and I go out to dinner. My mother-in-law vehemently disagrees. She thinks mothers shouldn't breastfeed in public. Who is right?*

A You have every right to breastfeed in public, but you don't have the right to put on a show, if you know what I mean. One key to breastfeeding in public is being discrete and showing respect for others. Simply choose what you wear with this in mind, and take along a baby blanket or a shawl. After a trial run or two, you might even invite your mother-in-law to join you.

DO BREASTFED BABIES GROW UP SMARTER?

Q *I recently read that breastfed babies grow up to be smarter in high school than babies who were bottle fed. Is this true? If so, can you tell me why?*

A You are probably referring to a study that was published on the Web site of the medical journal *Pediatrics*. Researchers in New Zealand tracked 1,265 newborns from birth to age 18, hoping to learn whether academic performance in high school was related to how children were fed as infants.

When compared to students who were bottle fed as infants, those who were breastfed for eight months or more scored significantly higher on the following:

- Tests of reading comprehension
- Tests of mathematical ability
- Tests of scholastic ability
- Teacher ratings in reading

When results were adjusted for social, family, and pregnancy differences, students who were breastfed still came out on top.

Why did breastfed babies fare so well in this study? The authors believe that certain fatty acids—those that play a crucial role in brain development and are only found in breast milk—may explain their findings.

FREEZING BREAST MILK FOR LATER USE IS EASY

Q *I'm breastfeeding our three-week-old daughter and have more than enough for her needs. I want to begin freezing the extra milk for her use after I return to work. Can you give me some advice about freezing breast milk to use weeks to months later?*

A Freezing breast milk for use weeks to months later is easy. The milk should be chilled in the refrigerator then frozen within 24 hours after it's expressed.

Breast milk can be stored in a self-defrosting refrigerator freezer for up to three or four months. Milk stored in a deep freezer at zero degrees Fahrenheit or less should be used within six months.

If you plan on freezing your milk in plastic bags, consider doubling the bags; they may split when thawing.

You may want to freeze your milk in 2–4 ounce portions for ease in thawing.

One way to thaw a container of frozen breast milk is to set it in a larger container full of warm water and slowly add warmer water until the milk is thawed.

After thawing is complete, gently swirl the container to mix the milk. Thawed milk should be kept in the refrigerator and used within 24 hours of thawing.

- Do not defrost breast milk by using boiling or very hot water.
- Do not defrost breast milk in a microwave oven.
- Do not refreeze previously frozen milk.

A further thought: During the eighteenth century, infants in Boston were often sent to live with wet nurses in the country. Wet nurses were in such demand that colonial newspapers carried ads such as the following:

> "A woman with a good breast of milk will take in a Nurse Child, about six miles from Boston." *Morning Chronicle* (Boston), April 6, 1780.

A wet nurse's qualifications included the following:

- A healthy appearance
- Strong moral character
- A consistent flow of high-quality breast milk.

The quality of a wet nurse's milk was believed to be related to her emotional makeup which, in turn, was related to her hair color. Blondes were thought to have volatile emotions, so their milk was more likely to be uneven in quality. Thus, brunettes—not blondes—were preferred as wet nurses.

IS BREASTFEEDING A RELIABLE CONTRACEPTIVE?

Q *I'll soon be a first-time, breastfeeding mother. After the baby is born, my husband and I would like to wait at least a year before trying to have another child. Can you tell me whether breastfeeding is a reliable contraceptive?*

A Studies in other cultures have shown that most mothers who are totally breastfeeding do not ovulate and, therefore, conceive, for up to a year or longer. Total breastfeeding means the baby relies completely on mom for nourishment and for all of his sucking needs.

This rest period in the reproductive cycle comes about because frequent nursing inhibits the release of hormones that normally stimulate ovulation and prepare the uterus for a new pregnancy.

However, this method often doesn't always work in Western society because the frequency of breastfeeding slacks off when babies start sleeping through the night and are introduced to solid foods.

If you wish to space out your children, don't rely on breastfeeding as a contraceptive. The wise thing to do is talk it over with your doctor.

A further thought: Firstborn children appear to be fortune's favorites. Firstborns are overrepresented in the following groups:

- Students in graduate and professional schools
- Students at the higher IQ levels
- National Merit and Rhodes Scholars

- Who's Who in America
- Individuals on *Time* covers
- U.S. presidents

IS BREASTFEEDING EASIER THE SECOND TIME AROUND?

Q *I stopped breastfeeding my first baby when she was about three weeks old, mainly because I didn't seem to have enough milk to satisfy her. I'm now seven months pregnant with my second baby and am hesitant to try breastfeeding again. Is it possible that breastfeeding is easier the second time around?*

A Many mothers share your experience with their first baby and decide not to try breastfeeding at all the second time around. However, a study done at the Royal Children's Hospital in Bristol, England, and published in the British medical journal *Lancet* suggests you should try again.

The study found that mothers who had the greatest difficulty in providing adequate amounts of milk after their first pregnancy were the very mothers who had the greatest increase in their ability to produce milk following their second pregnancy.

A further thought: A recent study suggests that if a new mother is having difficulty with breastfeeding, she should turn on some classical music. It works for cows and should work for humans.

In a study of 1,000 Holstein cattle at two dairies that exposed the cows to fast, slow, or no music from 5:00 A.M. to 5:00 P.M. every day for nine weeks, researchers found that cows hearing music such as Beethoven's Pastoral Symphony or Simon and Garfunkel's "Bridge Over Troubled Water" gave 3 percent more milk that those with no soundtrack.

Fast, high-pitched music actually caused a small decrease in milk production. These same researchers, by the way, are now studying the effects of music on the ability of chickens to lay eggs.

DOES BREASTFEEDING LOWER THE RISK OF BREAST CANCER?

Q *I've heard that breastfeeding can lower a woman's risk of developing breast cancer. Can you tell me if this is true?*

A Yes, it's true. Research has shown that women who breastfeed have a lower incidence of breast cancer. As an added bonus, the longer a woman nurses, the lower her risk of developing breast cancer.

IS PHENOBARBITAL SAFE FOR NURSING MOTHERS?

Q *I'm eight months pregnant and have been taking phenobarbital for epilepsy since I was five years old. The doctor said I would have to take it for life. Can you tell me whether phenobarbital passes through into breast milk? If so, will it harm my baby?*

A Lots of women taking phenobarbital for epilepsy have successfully breastfed their babies. By observing two simple precautions, there's no reason why you can't too.

Precaution #1: Women consuming phenobarbital during breast feeding should observe their infants for sedation.

Because phenobarbital does pass through into breast milk, a nursing baby ingests a small amount of the drug each time the baby is put to breast. In turn, the drug is absorbed in the baby's intestine and builds up in the blood.

Rarely, the level of phenobarbital may accumulate in the nursing baby's blood to the point that the baby's blood level may be as high as her mother's.

Since phenobarbital is a sedative, it may cause sedation or sleepiness. Should you have a concern, check with your baby's doctor for advice. The doctor may want to measure the phenobarbital level in your baby's blood just to be sure.

Precaution #2: Women consuming phenobarbital during breastfeeding should not abruptly stop nursing.

Because the level of phenobarbital in your baby's blood may equal or exceed yours, you should not abruptly stop nursing. Symptoms of drug withdrawal have been reported in nursing infants after abrupt weaning from mothers taking phenobarbital.

When you're ready to wean your baby, it's better to do it gradually. Then, the amount of phenobarbital in your baby's blood will slowly drop to a level safe for weaning.

DO NURSING BABIES HAVE MORE BOWEL MOVEMENTS, EVEN LATER ON?

Q *I've read that breastfed babies have more bowel movements than bottle fed babies. But how about later on, at say three to six months of age?*

A The same thing holds true at three months of age. In one study, the average breastfed baby at three months of age had 3.8 stools per day, compared to 1.3 stools and 2 stools per day for milk and soy-fed babies, respectively.

A further thought: Many factors influence a woman's decision to breastfeed. For instance:

- Catholic women tend to be more likely to breastfeed than Protestant women.
- Married women are more likely to breastfeed than single women.

- Women undergoing a cesarean section are less likely to breastfeed than women who deliver vaginally.
- College-educated women and women living in the western part of the United States are most likely to choose breastfeeding.
- Black women are less likely to breastfeed their babies than nonblack women.

Finally, a father's support is critical in the decision to breastfeed.

BREASTFEEDING AND HEAVY COFFEE DRINKING MAY NOT MIX

Q *Sometimes, my baby gets real fussy about an hour after breastfeeding and can't get back to sleep. This fussiness only seems to happen during the day. Could my heavy, day-time coffee drinking be causing it?*

A Normally, the amount of caffeine in breast milk after a mother drinks coffee is probably too low to be clinically significant. However, buildup may occur in an infant whose mother drinks moderate-to-heavy amounts of coffee.

Irritability and poor sleeping patterns have been observed in nursing infants during periods of heavy maternal use of caffeine. Try switching to decaffeinated coffee for a few days, and see what happens. If that's too big a step, try limiting your coffee intake to two or three cups a day.

A further thought: Mild to moderate coffee drinking during pregnancy doesn't harm the growing fetus. However, several studies have associated high coffee consumption (six to eight cups of coffee per day) with decreased fertility, increased incidence of miscarriage, and low birthweight. However, none of these studies separated the effects of caffeine from smoking or drinking alcohol, both of which are often associated with coffee drinking.

IS PROZAC SAFE FOR NURSING MOTHERS?

Q *When my daughter, Emily Ann, was born two months ago, it was the happiest day of my life. She weighed 8½ pounds and was 21 inches long. She latched on right in the delivery room and has been nursing ever since.*

Despite the good beginning, I came down with postpartum depression. Things got so bad that my doctor put me on Prozac, which helped a lot. But a week or so later and ever since, Emily Ann started acting colicky, crying out in pain for hours on end. Needless to say, most days both of us get very little sleep.

When I asked Emily Ann's pediatrician whether the Prozac could be at fault, she said Prozac had been around for several years and was safe for nursing babies.

When I asked my OB about the Prozac at my six-week checkup, he said he didn't know and to ask my pediatrician. I told him what my pediatrician had said, and he just shrugged his shoulders.

To make matters even worse, I recently weighed Emily Ann, and she is only a few ounces above her birthweight. Can you tell me please whether all of these things could be caused by the Prozac? I would gladly stop taking it if I knew it was harming my baby.

A It's not uncommon for new mothers to get depressed and require treatment with a drug such as Prozac. But your question adds a nursing baby to the picture. Is your baby also getting Prozac in the milk? If so, is it causing your baby's symptoms? Let's do a little detective work and see what we can learn.

Almost every physician's office, hospital, and pharmacy in the United States has a copy of the *Physicians'*

Desk Reference, commonly known as the PDR. For more than 50 years, the PDR has been considered the authority on prescription drugs.

The drug company that makes Prozac placed the following warning in the 2004 PDR:

> Because Prozac is excreted in human milk, nursing while on Prozac is not recommended.

This warning was placed in the PDR at the Food and Drug Administration's insistence, because experts had raised concerns about the safety for infants of nursing mothers taking Prozac. Now, we're getting somewhere.

One group of experts, the American Academy of Pediatrics (AAP), classifies Prozac as one of those drugs for which the effect on nursing infants is "unknown but may be of concern."

Prozac is excreted in breast milk and absorbed by the nursing baby, according to the AAP. Once the drug is in the baby's system, it can buildup to potentially harmful levels because it's eliminated slowly by the baby's relatively immature liver and kidneys.

As a result, there have been several published reports of colic, feeding and sleep disorders, and slow weight gain in nursing babies whose mothers were taking Prozac.

Sound familiar? By the way, the babies improved when their mothers stopped taking the drug.

The AAP has also raised concerns about the possible harmful effects of Prozac on the rapidly developing brains of infants whose mothers are taking the drug while nursing. Though this possibility needs further study, the FDA was concerned enough to advise the manufacturer of Prozac to revise its labeling to include the recommendation against its use by nursing mothers.

Where does this information leave concerned mothers like you?

Thomas Hale, Ph.D., is the author of the highly respected book, *Medications and Mothers' Milk*. He recommends that nursing mothers taking Prozac discontinue the drug and switch to an alternative medication if needed.

Current information on Zoloft and Paxil suggest these medications have difficulty entering breast milk, and more importantly, the infant. Thus, they may be preferred drugs over Prozac for the treatment of depression in breastfeeding mothers.

Take what you have learned from this discussion back to the doctor who prescribed Prozac for your depression, and ask him whether Zoloft or Paxil might be an adequate substitute.

Don't stop the Prozac abruptly without starting another drug. Your well-being is important too.

Bleeding concerns in infants

THE CIRCUMCISION THAT WON'T STOP BLEEDING

Q *My daughter recently gave birth to an apparently healthy baby boy. But several hours after he was circumcised, a nurse discovered his diaper was soaked with blood. They rushed him to a bigger hospital for intensive care. After some tests, he was diagnosed with hemophilia. Can you tell me what causes hemophilia? Does hemophilia run in families?*

A You've just described the most common way hemophilia presents in the newborn: the circumcision that won't stop bleeding.

Taking your second question first, we've known for hundreds of years that hemophilia runs in families. Fifteen hundred years ago, Jewish law did not allow a baby boy to be circumcised if two older brothers had bled to death after the procedure. So, even then, it was recognized that the brother of a male child with a bleeding problem was highly likely to have a similar condition.

In more recent times, hemophilia became widely known when it affected members of several European royal families. It all started with Prince Albert and Queen Victoria who, as it turns out, was a hemophilia carrier. They had nine children, including five girls. Two of the girls, Alice and Beatrice, were also carriers. When Alice and Beatrice married, they had three sons with hemophilia and three daughter carriers. The three daughter carriers eventually married into Russian, German, and Spanish royalty. All together, the three daughters produced five sons who had the disease.

Fast forward to the early 1980s. Hemophilia made headlines as one of the first human disorders for which the responsible genes had been identified and cloned (copied) in the laboratory.

At least 10 proteins called clotting factors in the blood must work in concert to make blood clot. A change in any of these factors can cause excessive bleeding. Two of these bleeding disorders are known as hemophilia A and hemophilia B.

Hemophilia A is caused by a defect in the clotting protein named Factor VIII. Hemophilia B is caused by a defect in Factor IX. Hemophilia A and B have similar symptoms and are inherited in the same way. So when most people talk about hemophilia, they are referring to either hemophilia A or hemophilia B.

Depending on the exact defect in the clotting factor gene, hemophilia can be mild, moderate, or severe. Because all those affected in a given family will have the same change in their Factor VIII or Factor IX gene, the disease usually has the same degree of severity in different members of the same family.

The genes involved in producing both Factor VIII and Factor IX are located on the X chromosome. If you remember, the sex chromosome makeup for females is XX and the sex chromosome makeup for males is XY. Hemophilia occurs almost exclusively in males because males only have one X chromosome. If that chromosome is carrying the abnormal gene responsible for Factors VIII or IX, then abnormal clotting results.

Females have two X chromosomes. If one of a female's X chromosomes is affected by the abnormal clotting gene and the other is not, she becomes a carrier. It only takes one normal X chromosome for normal clotting.

The chances are 50:50 that each son of a female carrier will have the disease, and 50:50 that each daughter of a carrier will be a carrier. These odds are the same for each pregnancy.

A genetic counselor will most likely meet with your daughter and her husband and give them much more information than I have mentioned here, including how to plan for future pregnancies.

VAGINAL BLEEDING IN THE NEWBORN

Q *The day after my daughter was born I noticed streaks of blood on her diaper. Our pediatrician said it was coming from her vagina and would stop in a few days, which it did. Can you explain why it happened?*

A It's not unusual to find small amounts of blood—actually, it's more like spotting—coming from a baby's vagina shortly after birth. Before birth, certain maternal hormones stimulate the baby's uterus. After birth, when the baby is no longer exposed to these hormones, she will often have a small amount of "withdrawal" bleeding. This bleeding is not uncomfortable and usually stops within a few days to a week or so.

D. Gary Benfield, M.D.

WHY IS THIS SIX-WEEK-OLD SUDDENLY SO SICK?

What do you do when your normally happy six-week-old wakes up one morning, warm to the touch and grumpy? In Jamie's case, she called her pediatrician, told him the story, then made an appointment for later that day. But when her daughter, Emma, started to shake and her eyes rolled back, Jamie called 9-1-1. Working swiftly, the paramedics found a vein and infused a dose of phenobarbital to control the seizure. Then they rushed both mother and baby to the nearest hospital.
The emergency room doctor carefully reviewed Emma's history:

- Jamie's pregnancy with Emma had been easier than expected.
- She saw her doctor regularly, ate all the right foods, and gave birth at home, assisted by a midwife.
- The only unusual incident was a mild episode of bleeding from Emma's healing navel at two weeks of age.
- Exclusively breastfed, Emma had gained weight nicely.

Following admission to the hospital, Emma suddenly turned pale and stopped breathing. Responding quickly, the code team started chest compressions and inserted a breathing tube and took control of her breathing.
Confused and nearly hysterical, her parents begged for answers. What could possibly have turned their daughter into this unresponsive child, kept alive with life support?
One of the doctors noticed a large hematoma on the back of Emma's head. Two of her IV sites were now oozing blood. Did she have a bleeding problem? Had she bled inside her head?

An emergency CAT scan answered their questions but offered little hope. A massive area of hemorrhage had formed between her skull and brain. And if that wasn't enough, she had also suffered a stroke.

What could cause so much bleeding? Had she been abused? Vitamin K deficiency can cause bleeding at this age. Could that be the problem?

Turning to the parents, the doctors asked about vitamin K. Did their daughter get the usual injection at birth?

"When the midwife asked about vitamin K, we refused," the parents said. "We had no idea it was so important."

Further tests confirmed the doctors' suspicion; vitamin K deficiency was the culprit.

In a sad and tearful meeting with their minister and all the doctors involved in Emma's care, her parents asked them to stop the respirator and let her go peacefully.

A further thought: This tragic story underscores why the American Academy of Pediatrics recommends an intramuscular, 1 milligram dose of vitamin K for all full-term newborns. An essential factor in blood clotting, vitamin K is normally low in breast milk. Without the recommended supplement, breastfed infants, especially, may become deficient, resulting in a bleeding problem sometime during the first eight months of life.

A warning bleed, such as oozing from a circumcision or a healing navel, often precedes a life-threatening hemorrhage. Unfortunately, because the warning bleed is often minor, it's usually ignored.

Given the nationwide increase in home deliveries and a growing reliance on alternative medicine, parents are playing Russian roulette with their babies' lives when they refuse them vitamin K.

This story was adapted from the June 1998 issue of *Contemporary Pediatrics*.

D. Gary Benfield, M.D.

Infant air travel

IS AIRTRAVEL SAFE FOR HEALTHY NEWBORNS?

Q My baby is due the last week in April, and, so far, everything is fine. The catch is my husband has accepted a promotion, which means moving to Florida. He is scheduled to start his new job on May 20, and we plan on flying down together with the baby. We have family in Tampa, so we have lots of support. We also have a place to live. Can you tell me whether it's safe for a three-week-old baby to fly? What about the risk of catching a cold or some other infection? Do the airlines have any restrictions on flying with a baby this age?

A We now know that healthy newborns are fit to fly. This fact has led most of the major airlines to remove all restrictions that formerly banned newborns from flying in the first few weeks of life. The restrictions were a throwback to the early days of flying when the aircraft were not pressurized, when oxygen was sometimes required during flights, and when little was known about newborn physiology and how infants would respond in flight.

As far as I know, no data suggest that newborns and infants are at increased risk of acquiring infectious diseases during air travel. However, debate about air quality in the aircraft cabin continues.

In recent years, to save money, airlines changed the method of supplying air to aircraft in flight. Under the old system, air was exchanged every few minutes. Fresh air was taken in from the outside and was virtually sterile, because no germs can live at 30,000 feet in the air. The outside air then passed through the hot engines and was cooled. This process is expensive.

Under the new system, half of the air in the cabin is recirculated and passed through sophisticated filters, making it virtually as germ-free as fresh air. But some experts question whether the filters eliminate all viruses. The consensus seems to be that the risk of acquiring an infection in-flight is small, but it does exist.

Parents have few options for protecting their infants from the risks of exposure to germs in flight. Certainly, if a nearby passenger is coughing and sneezing, you should ask to change seats.

Bring your own pillow and blankets; lately, many airlines exchange pillows ands blankets only when they are visibly soiled, sometimes once every few weeks.

After your baby is born and has been thoroughly evaluated, be sure to tell your baby's doctor about your plans and ask for advice. Also, to avoid any last minute delays at the airport, call your airline and tell them about your plans. Ask about their policies and procedures for flying with newborn infants.

A further thought: To minimize ear discomfort when flying, babies should be breastfed or bottle fed, or given something to suck on or drink during takeoff and landing. If a baby is asleep on takeoff, let her sleep. But when the plane starts descending, you might wake her up if she's asleep and offer her something to suck on or drink to keep her swallowing.

Preventing sudden infant death

> "The simple act of changing a baby's sleeping position from stomach to back has spared thousands of families the grief of losing a child."

IMPORTANT CHANGES IN GUIDELINES TO PREVENT SIDS

The American Academy of Pediatrics (AAP) has recently made some important changes in its guidelines to help prevent sudden infant death, or SIDS. Before we discuss these changes, however, let's define SIDS and review the AAP's role in trying to prevent it.

SIDS is the sudden death of an infant under one year of age, which remains unexplained after the following:

- Examining the death scene
- Reviewing the clinical history
- Performing a complete autopsy
- Investigating the case

Approximately 90 percent of all SIDS deaths occur during the first six months of life, most of them between two and four months of age. Most infants who die of SIDS die at home, usually while asleep, hence the terms *crib death* or *cot death*. What causes SIDS is still an unanswered question.

Fifteen years ago, doctors in many countries around the world had already begun to lower the incidence of SIDS by urging parents to put their babies to sleep on their backs. But doctors in the United States didn't joined in.

So when the AAP first advised pediatricians in 1992 to tell parents to put their babies to sleep on their backs, a lot of doctors ignored the advice, thinking it a silly idea.

Undaunted, the AAP went public in 1994 by launching the "Back to Sleep" campaign. As a result, the number of infant deaths caused by SIDS dropped from more than 5,000 in 1990 to about 2,600 in 1999, proving the doubters wrong.

The simple act of changing a baby's sleeping position from stomach to back has spared thousands of families the grief of losing a child.

Despite this impressive feat, SIDS still causes more infant deaths after the newborn period (first 28 days of life) than any disease. So now, in light of new research, the AAP has revised its guidelines to prevent SIDS, hoping to save even more lives. However, don't be surprised if the following changes bring out the doubters once again:

Walking the Baby Beat

- The AAP no longer recognizes sleeping on the side as a reasonable alternative to sleeping on the back. Studies have found that the side sleep position is unstable and increases the chances of the infant rolling onto her stomach. Every infant should sleep on her back at all times.
- Bed sharing is not recommended during sleep. Infants may be brought into bed for nursing or comforting, but should be returned to their own crib or bassinet when the parent is ready to return to sleep. However, growing evidence indicates that room sharing—infant sleeping in a crib in his parent's bedroom—is related to a reduced risk of SIDS. Thus the AAP recommends separate, but close by, infant sleeping.
- Research has shown a relationship between using a pacifier and a reduced risk of SIDS. So the AAP now recommends using a pacifier at nap time and at bedtime during the first year of life. However, once the infant falls asleep, if the pacifier falls out it should not be reinserted. The AAP believes the evidence that using a pacifier inhibits breastfeeding or causes later dental problems is not strong enough to discredit using a pacifier in this way.
- If a mother is breastfeeding, the AAP recommends delaying the introduction of a pacifier when putting a baby down to sleep until the infant is one month of age and breastfeeding is firmly established. If the infant refuses the pacifier, it should not be forced.

A further thought: All babies need "tummy time" when awake. This tummy position not only prevents flattening the back of a baby's head from too much time on her back, but it also helps strengthen her arms and shoulders when she begins pushing up to take in the wide world around her.

D. Gary Benfield, M.D.

BABIES NEED TUMMY TIME TOO

Q *I'd like to share a true story. After reading your column reminding parents of the new guidelines to place babies on their backs while sleeping, I shared it with my daughter. She not only knew about the guidelines, but had followed them religiously: My adorable six-week-old grandson had never been placed on his stomach, even when awake. When she took your advice and turned him on his stomach, he pushed himself up, looked around and giggled with delight. Perhaps doctors should remind parents that babies need time on their stomachs too.*

A Thank you for the reminder. When the Back-to-Sleep guidelines were first published, the American Academy of Pediatrics assumed that parents would place their babies on their stomachs when awake. No one anticipated that the fear of SIDS would lead some parents to keep their babies on their backs continuously. Your delightful experience confirms that babies need a certain amount of tummy time to push up and look around at the wide, wide world.

A further thought: During the second year of life, when toddlers discover that everything has a name, their vocabularies explode. By 18 months of age, a child will learn as many as 12 new words a day.

ISN'T SIDE SLEEPING FOR BABIES A GOOD COMPROMISE?

Q *I'm a nurse, and I work in a hospital nursery. I'm uncomfortable telling parents to place their babies on their backs; it seems too extreme. Isn't side sleeping a good compromise?*

A No. Here's what research shows regarding side sleeping:

- A baby who sleeps on his side is at twice the risk of SIDS as a baby who sleeps on his back.
- The side position is unstable; a baby can easily roll onto her stomach.
- Parents whose doctors recommend that their babies only sleep on their backs are most likely to place their infants on their backs.
- Parents whose doctors recommend a side position are least likely to place their babies on their backs.

Side sleeping is now unacceptable in light of the American Academy of Pediatrics (AAP) revised guidelines to prevent SIDS.

A further thought: The AAP also advises parents not to put their babies to sleep on soft bedding. The theory here is that some babies have a delay in their brains' arousal mechanisms. This means that some babies don't arouse when their faces get nuzzled under a quilt or against a soft mattress, resulting in suffocation. Here's what the AAP advises about bedding:

- Make sure your baby sleeps on a firm mattress.
- Don't use fluffy blankets or comforters under the baby.
- Don't let your baby sleep on a waterbed, sheepskin, a pillow, or other soft materials.
- When your baby is very young, don't place soft stuffed toys or pillows in the crib; these soft materials increase the risk of smothering.

Growth and development after birth

WILL OUR 14-MONTH-OLD EVER WALK?

Q *My son sat up at five months and said "da-da" at eight. But at 14 months, he refuses to walk. He's perfectly content* to roam the house on his hands and knees. Meanwhile, the other neighborhood children his age all walk. One child even walked at 11 months. Do we have the first kid in history who will never learn to walk?

A Put away those books that say babies sit up at six months, blurt out "ma-ma" and "da-da" by nine months, and start walking at a year. There's no need to panic just because your son isn't keeping up with the junior Joneses. The leap from crawling to walking can happen anytime from 9 to 17 months. The point isn't to walk for its own sake but to get somewhere. And your son is doing that perfectly well by crawling.

If you are still concerned, ask your son's doctor what she or he thinks.

FATHER PRAYS FOR LEFT-HANDED SON

Q My husband prays every night that our three-month-old son will grow up and become a left-handed pitcher for the Cleveland Indians. Is there anything we can do to safely encourage our son to use his left hand?

A We don't fully understand what makes a person right- or left-handed. But most experts agree it's a mistake to force a child to use a certain hand, because right- or left-handedness seems to be programmed into our brains from birth.

A further thought: The year 1999 marked the first time that a full one-third of all U.S. births were to unwed mothers. Of approximately 4 million births, 1,308,560 were to unwed mothers, the highest number ever recorded up until that time.

Studies show that one of the reasons we are reluctant to deal with this disgraceful statistic is that the American public typically views teen childbearing and unwed childbearing as one and the same. But most unwed mothers are in their twenties, not in their teens.

EIGHT-MONTH-OLD HAS NO TEETH

Q *Our eight-month-old doesn't have any teeth. Can you tell me if this is normal?*

A The first tooth usually appears at about six months of age. However, the range of normal varies from four to twelve months. As long as your baby is growing and developing normally, the later arrival of teeth is not a cause for concern.

TOE-SUCKING SON HAS PARENTS WORRIED

Q *My husband and I are concerned about our three-year-old son's behavior. He will take off his shoes and socks and put his big toe in his mouth, mostly at home, but sometimes in public. He has never sucked his thumb and did not particularly like a pacifier. He has always preferred his toes.*

We have tried everything our doctor has suggested to break him of this habit, but nothing works. We even painted his toenails with a nasty-tasting solution, but it didn't help. Can you offer any suggestions?

A Lots of children comfort themselves when anxious, stressed, or bored by sucking their thumb or clinging to a favorite object. But your resourceful son has taken the art of relaxing to a new level. He not only gets attention, but he embarrasses his parents as well.

To make sure the habit isn't affecting the alignment of his teeth, make an appointment with your dentist to have your son's teeth checked. If the dentist is concerned, he may recommend installing a device in your son's mouth to prevent the toe from putting pressure on the teeth.

An added benefit of such a device is that it also makes placing the toe into the mouth unpleasant. This fact, in itself, might help your son give up the habit.

If your son's behavior is not affecting his teeth, you should ask yourselves, what's all the fuss about? Exerting pressure on him to stop sucking his toe seems to be doing more harm than good. I suspect that if you and your husband could mutually agree to ignore his behavior, peer pressure from outside the home will eventually help him stop.

NO CRAWLING FOR THIS CHILD

Q *Our 14-month-old daughter seemed to skip the crawling stage and started pulling up to furniture and then to walking. Is this unusual?*

A Experts say that 10 to 15 percent of children walk without ever having crawled. Some of these children also walk earlier than expected. There's no need for concern.

THREE-MONTH-OLD DOESN'T CRY MUCH

Q *Our 12 week-old daughter seems quite healthy, but she doesn't cry more than 15 to 30 minutes a day. I'm curious. Can you tell me how much babies this age normally cry?*

A One of America's best-known pediatricians, T. Berry Brazelton, M.D., researched your question some 35 years ago. He found that at two weeks of age the average crying time was nearly two hours per day, increasing to nearly three hours at six weeks and then declining to about one hour at 12 weeks. Don't worry about your daughter's "below-average" crying time. Sounds like she's just a laid-back child.

WHY IS THIS CHILD SUCH A DADDY'S GIRL?

Q *Our only child is 10 months old, and we love her very much. Our pediatrician says she's the picture of good health, but one thing bothers me: When my husband comes into the room, she cries and reaches out for him, even if I'm holding her or playing with her at the time.*
Can you tell me whether her behavior is normal? I hate to admit it, but I'm feeling jealous and don't know what to think. Am I blowing things out of proportion or should I be concerned?

A Most infants enjoy being alone with either parent. But when both parents are in the room, they often pick one parent they prefer to be with. Usually they choose their mother, but right now, temporarily, your daughter has picked her father.

Just as babies learn to relate more to fathers in time, your daughter will soon begin to relate more to you. I suggest you try to relax and take your daughter's current preference in stride. This too shall pass.

WHEN A FIVE-MONTH-OLD DROOLS AND BLOWS BUBBLES

Q *Our five-month-old has started drooling and blowing bubbles. Does this behavior mean a tooth is coming in? Can you tell me why infants drool?*

A Drooling is caused by an increased flow of saliva that often heralds the appearance of a new tooth. Saliva is produced in the salivary glands. The submandibular gland is located under the chin, the sublingual gland is under the tongue, and the parotid glands are located in front of the ears.

The increased flow of saliva has several important functions:

- It seems to sooth the baby's tender gums.
- It softens and moistens food once solid foods are started.
- It keeps the mouth moist and makes it easier to swallow.
- It washes away residual food and protects against tooth decay.

A further thought: Saliva is also a natural antacid. It neutralizes stomach acid and aids digestion.

WILL OUR 10-MONTH-OLD WALK SOONER WEARING SHOES?

Q *My husband and I disagree about shoes for our 10-month-old son. I think he will learn to walk sooner if we put him in shoes. My husband feels we should wait, and let him learn to walk without shoes. What do you think?*

A In general, shoes don't help a child learn to walk sooner. Most foot experts believe that shoes are unnecessary until after a child has learned to walk. When buying shoes for a toddler, it's important to select a store that employs well-trained salespersons you can trust.

WHEN TO INTRODUCE INFANTS TO PICTURE BOOKS

Q *I began reading to my four-month old almost from the day she was born. Recently, I introduced her to picture books. My* *problem is she still doesn't seem all that interested. Am I doing something wrong, or is there possibly, God forbid, something amiss with her?*

A I doubt that you are doing something wrong, or that there is something wrong with your baby. In the first six months of life, a baby's main interest is people, not objects. By the age of six months, increased visual acuity, the ability to sit straighter and the ability to focus their attention helps babies expand their interests. They start to reach out to objects and begin smiling and waving their arms and legs in response to the pictures in books.

Try putting the picture books aside temporarily. Instead, take her in your arms, and act out your own made-up stories. My guess is she will love it. Be careful not to overload her. Try it for a few minutes, two or three times a day. Then, reintroduce her to picture books at six months of age. Chances are she will then become interested.

HOW INFANTS FEEL ABOUT STRANGERS

Q *When my daughter was three months old, she broke out into a body-wiggling smile every time a stranger approached and was willing to smile and make noises at her. Now that she's five months old, she seems to have changed her mind.*

When the doctor recently came near her, she eyed him suspiciously, began to shriek, and cried long after the exam was over. Is this another stage she's going through, or should I be concerned?

A Most children your daughter's age become sensitive about strangers and new places between five and six months of age. Don't be concerned. Try making a special effort to reassure her when among new people or places. Most children outgrow stranger anxiety by the end of the first year.

A further thought: A nearly fatal misjudgment marked Pablo Picasso's birth. Thinking him stillborn, the midwife abandoned him on a table. But his uncle, a cigar-smoking physician, revived him with a blast of smoke-filled air into his lungs, according to *Isaac Asimov's Book of Facts.*

THE DAD DIFFERENCE IN CHILD DEVELOPMENT

Q *Are there things that only fathers can give their children growing up?*

A Before I answer your question, it might be helpful, even comforting, to list some of the ways mothers and father are similar:

- In general, men and women are both inclined emotionally to nurture their children. The problem is they are not similarly prepared or supported by society—or their own families—to do so. Given equal experience and support, no evidence shows that one gender excels over the other as parents.
- The desire to feel emotionally connected to one's child is the same for men and women.
- Fathers and mothers are equally able to interpret their child's behavior and respond appropriately.
- Fathers and mothers are equally anxious about leaving their child in the care of someone else.
- Single parenting is strikingly similar for men and women.

Even though mothers and fathers share these similarities, we also know fathers do not mother and, clearly, mothers do not father. This observation leads to your question, "Are there things that only fathers can give their children?"

Walking the Baby Beat

In his very important book, *Fatherneed,* Kyle D. Pruett, M.D., points out that researchers have just begun to understand the dad differences in child development. So don't take anything I say as the final answer.

Studies show that infants who have benefited from highly involved dads during the first two years of life tend to share the following characteristics:

- They are more secure in exploring the world around them.
- They tend to be more curious and less hesitant or fearful, especially when confronted by new or unusual situations.
- By the time these children are ready for school, they tend to have greater tolerance for stress and frustration, a quality that will stand them in good stead in a class with 29 other kids and one very busy teacher.

Incidentally, Pruett's own mother, a veteran teacher with more than 50 years in elementary education, claims she can pick out the "well-fathered" kids in her classes by their self-confidence and willingness to try new things.

When preschoolers of highly involved dads were compared to preschoolers with less-involved fathers, children of the dad-involved group had higher levels of verbal skills. Research also shows that involved, but overly strict fathers can lead to more, not fewer, school problems, such as being less sociable and taking less initiative. Overly strict limit setting by fathers has its own limitations.

Hardly any behavior in boys and girls is more valued by parents than self-control. Studies show that children with positively involved fathers display less impulsivity and more self-control than children with negatively involved fathers.

One highly regarded study found that positive paternal engagement, for boys and for girls, is closely associated with the following:

- A lower incidence of acting out, disruptive behavior, depression, sadness, and lying
- Getting along well with others, and being responsible
- Boys having fewer school behavioral problems
- Girls having more cheerful and happy interchanges, greater capacity for positive self-involvement, and greater willingness to try new things

The father factor in child development also exerts its influence indirectly. For instance, when a mother feels supported by the father, she tends to be more patient, flexible, emotionally responsive, and available to her children.

Affectionate and caring fathering is also associated with more positive sibling interactions, suggesting that father's involvement has significant indirect effects on the entire family.

In the end, mothers and fathers share many more nurturing behaviors than they do not, and they reinforce these behaviors in each other. This effect is what seems to matter most to children.

WHY WON'T THIS SEVEN-MONTH-OLD EAT BABY FOOD?

Q *Our daughter is seven months old and growing like a weed, but she still refuses to eat baby food. We have tried almost daily since she was four months old, but all she does is push out her tongue. If we do get some food in her mouth, she gags. Any suggestions?*

A Let's take a deep breath and think this situation through. Before six months of age, babies are designed to suck, not chew. They have a tongue-thrust reflex that causes the tongue to automatically protrude when a substance like baby food is placed on the tongue.

Between four and six months, this reflex usually starts to fade, then disappears. Also, before six months of age, infants usually can't coordinate their tongues and swallowing movements for solid foods. An added sign that babies were not designed for the early introduction of solid foods is that teeth seldom appear before six or seven months of age.

You tried to introduce solid foods almost daily since your daughter was four months of age, and she resisted. Those daily battles perhaps prolonged her tongue-thrusting reflex and her inability to coordinate her swallowing movements for solid foods. Add to these factors a touch of stubbornness, and you have a stand-off.

My advice?

- Step back and relax.
- Accept your daughter for the unique person that she is.
- For the next week or two, only offer her formula.
- Then gradually reintroduce baby food by placing some banana on your finger to see if she will suck it down.
- If she smiles and seems to like it, gradually increase the amount, placing a glob toward the middle of her tongue.
- After she gets used to the new taste and texture of solids, progress from a fingertip-full, to a half teaspoonful, to a teaspoonful, then to a tablespoonful.
- Don't expect her to eat the same amount each day. She may eventually take a whole jar one day, but only a tablespoonful the next.

A further thought: It's wise to introduce each new food one at a time rather than several foods mixed together. In case a baby is allergic to, or dislikes a food, offering a single food makes it easier to identify the culprit.

WHY DO BABIES SLEEP DIFFERENTLY THAN ADULTS?

Q *My husband and I have been reading a lot about how babies and adults sleep, but it gets very confusing. Can you explain the difference between REM and non-REM sleep and why it helps for learning how babies sleep? At what age do most babies sleep through the night?*

A Warning: My answer contains a lot of information to retain with just one reading. However, if you read it through two or three times, it will all make sense. I guarantee it.

During rapid eye movement or REM sleep, we exercise our brain by dreaming while our eyes move beneath our closed lids, as if we are watching our dreams. We may also startle, twitch our face, make jerking movements with our hands and feet, and tend to wake up more easily. So you see, we do not sleep soundly during REM sleep.

Non-REM sleep consists of four phases:

- Drowsiness
- Light sleep
- Deep sleep
- Very deep sleep

As we progress from drowsiness to deepest sleep, we become less and less active. Our breathing slows and becomes very quiet. In deepest sleep, we are virtually motionless. We do very little, if any, dreaming during non-REM sleep.

Now, let's compare how adults and babies sleep.

Adults cycle through all four of the non-REM phases of sleep before entering REM sleep and start dreaming as follows:

- Drowsiness
- Light sleep

- Deep sleep
- Very deep sleep
- REM sleep

The typical adult passes back and forth throughout the night between REM and non-REM sleep, spending about six hours in deep sleep and two hours in active REM sleep.

Babies, on the other hand, fall asleep in the following order:

- Drowsiness
- REM sleep
- Light sleep
- Deep sleep
- Very deep sleep

Unlike adults, babies only sleep for three to four hours at a stretch, evenly spaced between feedings, throughout the day and night. Also, unlike adults, each of these sleep periods is divided almost equally between REM and non-REM sleep. Let's summarize these differences before moving ahead:

- Unlike adults, babies enter sleep through REM sleep.
- Unlike adults, sleep periods are shorter for babies and continue around the clock.
- Babies experience as much REM sleep in each sleeping period as adults do during a whole night of sleep. Thus babies exercise their brains more while sleeping, are more vulnerable for waking up, and are more vulnerable for difficulty getting back to sleep.
- Adults sleep 6–8 hours each night while babies sleep from 16–18 hours each day and night.

Now, let's apply what we've learned.

Adults can go directly from wakefulness into a state of deep sleep rather quickly, but babies can't.

Babies first go through a period of REM sleep before entering deep sleep.

For example, it's time to put baby to bed. Her eyes close completely, but her eyelids continue to flutter, her breathing is still irregular, and she may startle and twitch and show fleeting smiles. You gently place her in the crib and quietly creep away, but she wakes up. That's because she was still in REM sleep when you put her down.

You pick her up and relax in a rocking chair. Soon her grimaces and twitches stop; her breathing becomes more regular and shallow; her muscles relax. Her arms and legs dangle limply, a sign of deep, non-REM sleep. Now you can put her down and sneak away; your baby is finally asleep.

An hour or so later, your baby begins to squirm. She tosses a bit, her eyelids flutter, she breathes irregularly, and her muscles tighten. She is reentering REM sleep and probably dreaming.

During this vulnerable period, many babies awaken if any upsetting stimulus occurs. Over the next 10 minutes baby drifts through this light sleep period and descends back into deep sleep.

For the rest of the night? Not yet. Another hour passes and she reenters REM sleep, another vulnerable period occurs, and this time she awakens and then wakes you up.

Scientists believe that REM sleep is good for babies because it provides mental exercise. Dreaming during REM sleep provides visual images for baby's brain, stimulating its development.

But when will your baby sleep through the night?

The age at which babies go to sleep easily and stay asleep for extended periods of time varies widely. In the first three months, a baby's sleep habits resemble her feedings: small frequent feedings, short frequent naps.

After three months of age, most babies are awake for longer stretches during the day, and some may sleep for five-hour stretches, the medical definition of "sleeping through the night."

This achievement marks the beginning of a gradual shift toward the adult pattern of going to sleep: cycling through the non-REM phases of sleep before entering REM sleep. By the age of three, only one-third or less of total sleep time is spent in REM sleep.

By the way, feeding babies solid foods at bedtime rarely helps them sleep longer, as you might guess from what we've learned.

IS THIS BABY'S SLEEPING BEHAVIOR ABNORMAL?

Q *My mother has me all confused and upset. She says there's something wrong with my baby because he sometimes twitches, jerks, and moves his eyes when asleep. Is this unusual behavior? If so, what should I do about it?*

A I doubt that anything is wrong with your baby. The movements are probably occurring when he is dreaming, during rapid eye movement (REM) sleep. To be sure, ask your doctor.

GIVING TEMPERAMENT ITS DUE

Q *Our three-year-old son has always been an easy child. As a baby, he loved to be held, slept between feedings, and rarely cried. He sat up at six months, walked at a year, and eagerly adjusted to strangers. As a result, my husband and I thought parenting was relatively easy.*

But all that changed seven months ago when our daughter was born. Unlike her brother, she responds to cuddling or playful attempts to get her to smile by frantically waving her arms or arching her back and crying. A frequent spitter, it's almost like she's trying to shut us out. How can two children be so different? Can you explain why what seemed to work for our son doesn't work for our daughter?

A Most parents don't recognize the importance of temperament until after their second child is born. By temperament we mean the style a child uses to interact with the world.

Some infants are extremely active, moving their arms and legs incessantly. Others are tranquil. Some children explore their environment eagerly for great lengths of time. Others do not. Some infants respond warmly to people. Others fuss and fret. All of these behavioral styles represent a child's temperament. Your task is to watch and listen for each child's particular style, not to compare one child to the other.

Take your daughter, for example, we might call her a hypersensitive baby. When approached with loving affection, every system in her body seems to say, "I am overloaded."

Try introducing one new experience at a time—speak softly or look her in the face or rock her gently—but only try one. Learning to take in and absorb all three might be too much to ask. By introducing one new stimulus at a time, you can gradually teach her to take in the world, not shut it out.

Experts believe genes and experience each contribute about 50 percent to a child's temperament. However, the extent to which parents can mold a child's behavior depends, in part, on the "match" or "fit" between the child's temperament and that of her parents.

For instance, an easy-going parent may have a calming effect on a difficult child, eventually encouraging more appropriate behavior. On the other hand, a high-strung parent may withdraw from the child or become critical and punish her, making the child even more difficult to parent.

COPING WITH COLIC

Talking to myself about colicky babies.

  I: What is colic, anyway?
Me: It depends on whom you ask. No two experts agree on one definition.

Walking the Baby Beat

I: Is that your sly way of saying you don't know?
Me: Not exactly. It's my way of saying there is no generally accepted definition.
I: Ok. Stop hedging. Give it your best shot.
Me: Colic can be defined as crying during the first three months of life for three or more hours a day on three or more days a week in infants who are otherwise healthy.
I: That's a mouthful. But don't babies normally cry more during the first three months of life?
Me: That's true.
I: What am I missing here? Why are some babies labeled as colicky and others not?
Me: Good question. It depends on how upset the parents get and whether they bring it up to their doctor.
I: Are you saying that colic involves upset babies and upset parents?
Me: That's right. It's hard for any parent to calmly respond, night after night, to a screaming baby whose flushed face, tense belly, and stiffened arms and legs suggests intense pain.
I: You mean holding and walking the baby, offering a pacifier, rocking the child; none of these tricks seems to help?
Me: That's often true. Then the next morning someone, usually the mother, is too exhausted to face the day.
I: Why do you suppose colic seems to improve around three months of age?
Me: One theory says that around three months most babies learn to soothe themselves and interact more with their caregivers. Then the colic improves.
I: Are you saying colic ends when a baby's development reaches a certain stage?
Me: Something like that.
I: So if parents can see their infant's colic as a temporary kind of behavior, they may feel less overwhelmed knowing it will pass?

Me: That attitude certainly helps. Then parents can sit down with their doctor and calmly put a plan together. That way, one parent doesn't have to bear the burden alone.
I: So a sense of optimism helps?
Me: Let me put it this way: A pessimistic attitude usually leads to failure.
I: One final question: Don't parents sometimes get angry when their baby won't stop crying?
Me: That's true. In fact, some parents get so angry that they feel like shaking their baby.
I: Isn't that dangerous?
Me: Of course, knucklehead; shaking a baby is extremely dangerous. It can cause brain bleeds and broken bones. Seriously, when parents feel their anger coming on, they need to take a break and get help immediately.

Parenting

WHEN DOES LOVE BEGIN?

Q *After my baby was born, I checked her over from head to toe then gave her up and fell asleep, exhausted. The next morning, I noticed that I didn't feel particularly close to my baby. But later that evening, everything changed when I looked into her eyes. At that moment, I suddenly realized I had the most perfect, most gorgeous, most responsive baby in the world. For the first time I felt an incredible love for my baby.*

My girlfriends all say they first experienced this kind of feeling either during their pregnancies or at the moment of birth. Was my experience unusual? Does it mean I love my baby less?

Walking the Baby Beat

A Your experience is not unusual, and it doesn't at all suggest that you love your baby less. The British pediatrician, Aidian MacFarlane, and his associates asked 97 mothers, "When did you first feel love for your baby?" They responded this way:

- During pregnancy   41 percent
- At birth   24 percent
- First week   27 percent
- After the first week 8 percent

Each parent develops love for a new baby in a different way and at a different pace.

Emotional issues that go unresolved during pregnancy will often surface when a baby is born and delay feelings of love for the baby.

Take, for example, the mother who plans to return to work after her pregnancy leave is over. Even before her baby is born, she may feel conflicted over becoming too attached to the baby and then returning to work full-time. Her conflict may also influence her decision to breastfeed. Until her conflict is acknowledged and explored, say with her baby's pediatrician, she may have difficulty developing a deep and sustained bond with her baby.

Some birthing practices can also delay feelings of love for a baby. They include the following:

- Whisking the healthy baby away from its parents in the first few minutes after birth
- Placing the healthy infant under a warmer instead of using skin-to-skin contact to keep the baby warm
- Treating the baby's eyes with antibiotic ointment before mom has had a chance to see them
- Being surrounded by the hustle and bustle of so many strangers in the birthing room

Quiet time alone with their baby helps parents fall in love, not only with their baby, but with each other all over again.

A further thought: Falling in love may occur in a single, magical moment. Staying in love is a long-term process that demands lots of work.

HELPING A CHILD ADJUST TO A NEW SIBLING

Q *My wife just learned that she's pregnant. Can you suggest how we might help our eight-year-old daughter adjust to the new baby?*

A Helping an eight-year-old adjust to a new baby should be relatively easy. The main ingredients are finding the time and making a commitment.

Let's divide the process into three parts:

- Preparation
- Explanation
- Participation

Preparation begins with deciding how and when to tell your daughter about the baby. An eight-year-old should probably be told before or as soon as you begin telling friends and relatives.

If your hospital offers a sibling visitation program, consider taking her to see where the babies are born and where she will visit her mother and the new baby.

Explanation begins with honesty. If you and your wife haven't already done so, consider explaining the basic facts about conception and pregnancy so she can understand where babies come from and how she relates to the new baby.

Walking the Baby Beat

Several excellent books are available to not only help with your explanation, but to keep you from feeling embarrassed. Explanations such as babies are delivered by the stork may seem cute, but won't help an eight-year-old understand or accept the new situation.

Participation should be the easiest part. Children your daughter's age are usually eager to help. The three of you can fix up the baby's bedroom, pick out furniture, and go shopping for baby clothes. If it's necessary to move your daughter to another bedroom, make the move before the baby is born.

After the baby is born, you can take your daughter to the hospital to welcome the new baby and to feel like she's part of your expanding family. Later, you and your wife can involve her in supervised baby care activities.

Throughout your wife's pregnancy and especially after the baby is born, it's important for both you and your wife to stay involved in your daughter's activities and to pay attention to her needs. Spend some time with her each day, using the time to help her feel special and loved.

A further thought: American women consume an average of four to five different drugs during pregnancy. The majority of these drugs have never been tested for fetal effects, which are often discovered later.

WHEN A 15-MONTH-OLD URINATES IN THE BATH WATER

Q *My 15-month-old sometimes urinates in his bath. Obviously it isn't the most sanitary thing, but how upset should I be about it? Should I run him a new bath? And what about his tub toys?*

A I checked the published baby wizards, Drs. Spock, Brazelton, and Sears, but they have not addressed your question. So I turned to a dear friend who has raised two grown boys, my 83-year-old mother. Listen in on our telephone conversation.

"Hi mom, I need you help."
"What's wrong, Gary? Is someone sick?"
"Mom, we're fine. Will you help me answer a mother's question?"
"I don't know, Gary. Aren't you the doctor?"
"Yes mom. But I value your experience."
"How can I help?"
"Mom, when Eric and I were around 15 months old, did we ever urinate in our bath water?"
"I don't remember you boys doing something like that!"
"We didn't pee in the tub?"
"Not that I remember. I always put you on the potty before your bath."
"On the potty at 15 months?"
"That's right. You were potty trained by the time you started walking, at least the bladder part."
"But Mom, parents today don't potty train their kids that early."
"I know they don't, but back then we used cloth diapers. The sooner you were potty trained, the fewer diapers to wash."
"Well, suppose I had urinated in my bath water. What would you have done?"
"I would probably just laugh and ignore it."
"Laugh and ignore it?"
"That's right. It's kind of natural, you know."
"How about my toys. What would you have done with them?"
"Now Gary, you boys never had toys in the bath water. Getting a bath was all business."
"All business?"
"Oh, we played and splashed around. But you never had toys in the tub. Look, you tell that mother just put your son on the potty before he gets a bath. Forget the toys.

Walking the Baby Beat

Splash around and have a good time, but get it over with. If he pees in the tub, laugh about it and finish up."

"Mom, you're wonderful."

"Thank you, sweetheart. How are the girls?"

A further thought: While on the phone, our conversation soon turned to spanking. Mom said the only time she really spanked me was when I was about three. I wanted something and she told me I couldn't have it. So I threw myself on the floor and started screaming. She picked me up, paddled my butt, and said not to do that again. I never did. "You've got to correct these children," she said. "That's just part of training. You have to have discipline."

Mom passed away on August 25, 2005, at the age of 90.

SHOULD FATHERS SHARE IN THEIR BABIES' CARE?

Q *Some of the guys at work are ribbing me because I change our daughter's diapers, give her a bottle at night, and generally share in her care with my wife. Their reaction has me wondering: Am I doing the right thing?*

A Research shows that when fathers are involved in their babies' care, their babies benefit enormously. For example, teenagers whose fathers were involved with them as infants tend to have higher IQs, a greater sense of humor, longer attention spans, more eagerness for learning, and are more resistant to peer pressure than teens of uninvolved fathers. Seems to me, you're on the right track, regardless of what your co-workers think.

A further thought: This country's most famous baby doctor, Benjamin Spock, M.D., died in 1997 at the age of 94. He began his best-selling book, *Baby and Child Care,* by offering this advice to parents:

"Trust yourself, you know more than you think you do."

D. Gary Benfield, M.D.

"READ ME A STORY"

Q *It seems that everywhere I turn someone is urging parents to read to their children. Even Hillary Clinton has gotten into the act. Can you explain why reading to my children is so important?*

A According to experts, such as the American Academy of Pediatrics, America is in a reading crisis. Far too many children are growing up without the reading skills they need to succeed in school and life. Recent studies reveal that:

- More than 40 percent of fourth graders read below grade level.
- Children ages 9 to 14 spend more than 20 percent of their waking hours watching television, but only 1 percent of waking time reading.
- Only 50 percent of parents routinely read to their infants and toddlers.

The AAP recommends that pediatricians prescribe reading to children beginning at six months of age. In this way, as these children grow, they will not only learn words and concepts but, more important, they will get excited about books and enjoy reading.

Something magical happens when a child crawls up on the lap of a parent or grandparent and says, "Please read me a story." The intimacy of sharing books and stories helps strengthen the emotional bond between adult and child. I still remember how thrilled I was to sit on my grandfather's knee reading stories.

Research also shows that reading to children stimulates the growth of a baby's brain. When a child is born, that area of the brain known as the brain stem—which controls our reflexes, breathing, and heart rate—is already wired.

In the higher centers of the brain, however, neural circuits are primitive at best; the vast majority of the 1,000

Walking the Baby Beat

trillion connections that the newborn's billions of neurons will eventually make are therefore determined by early experience.

Reading, laughing, cooing, and hugging are some of the more important early experiences that will help reinforce and permanently wire all those tentative connections.

Here are some things a baby's parents can do to help:

- Set aside time each day for reading. Make it part of your routine.
- Don't wait until six months of age to begin reading to your baby. Start right away, but only for a few minutes at a time.
- Recite nursery rhymes and sing songs. Rhymes help develop a young child's ear for language.
- Point to things in picture books and name them. As your child learns to talk, ask her to "point and say."

A further thought: Babies are born with their brains primed to learn. But they can't do it alone.

BABIES NEED PARENTS' ATTENTION, NOT JUST GAMES AND TOYS

Q *I'm an insecure first-time mother who wants to get her three-week-old son off to a good start. Can you recommend some games and toys for my baby?*

A By now, you probably know the difference between your son's cry for food and his cry for comfort. You are learning a lot each day, but your baby is learning much more. Every laugh, every song and peek-a-boo sets off messages to his brain, laying a framework for what could someday be a love of reading or a gift for making friends.

Wise parents have always known instinctively that young children need lots of attention from the significant adults in their lives. You don't need to go out and spend a small fortune on toys and games to give your son a good start. What you do need to do is to take advantage of your baby's natural curiosity.

Your baby is a learning machine: Everything interests him. Your voice, the sound of the washing machine, Celine Dion singing on the stereo, shadows on the wall are all fascinating to an infant.

Simple activities, such as cuddling and rocking a baby, stimulate growth. Games such as peek-a-boo teach babies about face-to-face communication. And, talking baby talk—the babbling known as parentese—teaches verbal interaction.

Studies have shown that babies who are hugged often and feel loved and cared for are much more likely to grow up confident and optimistic.

Games and toys for your baby? You and your son's father have them right at your fingertips.

P.S. If you must buy something, pick up several baby books and start reading to your son every day. Better yet, crank up your imagination and make up your own stories.

A further thought: By two weeks of age, a baby will know her father's voice and can distinguish his from other male voices. By four weeks of age, a baby will respond differently to each of her parents and to strangers.

THESE PARENTS STILL READ ALOUD TO THEIR SIX-YEAR-OLD

Q *My husband and I have read aloud to our six-year-old son almost daily since he was born, and he still loves it. After dinner, he picks out the story, and one of us reads to him while the other does the dishes. My problem is my mother says our son is getting too old for that sort of thing. She thinks he should spend the time reading to himself. What do you think?*

A These days, few American families follow a routine like the one you've described. Treasure it, and don't stop reading to your son until he asks you to.

CHOOSING YOUR BABY'S FIRST SITTER

Q My baby is due in two weeks, and I'm trying to plan ahead. We don't have family help nearby. Can you recommend how to go about finding a capable baby-sitter?

I also want to start a file of information about our baby's health. Can you tell me what kinds of information to include?

A Finding a reliable baby-sitter can be time consuming, but it's worth the effort. Start by asking your friends and neighbors for recommendations. Interview each candidate in person and with your baby present. Be sure to ask about each candidate's experience and ask for references.

If you feel comfortable with a particular candidate, let her hold your baby so you can see how she handles him. When it's all said and done, give your top choice a trial run with your baby while you're at home.

When you leave your baby with a sitter, give her a list of emergency phone numbers, including those where you and a trusted neighbor can be reached if problems arise. Establish clear guidelines about what to do in an emergency. Make sure she knows how to handle a child who is choking or not breathing.

Here's a list of medical information about your baby's health that all new parents should keep in a folder for future use:

- Name, address, and phone number of your baby's physician
- Immunizations, including dates administered
- Your child's height and weight at each doctor visit

- Screening test results (vision, hearing, and other aspects of your child's health)
- Hospitalizations (dates, illnesses, and treatments)
- Family medical history of any diseases that run in your extended family

A further thought: In today's managed care climate, first-time parents may have difficulty finding a pediatrician. Here are a few tips to help make your search easier:

- Start before your baby is born by asking your insurance company for a list of their pediatrician providers.
- Then ask your obstetrician to recommend two or three from the list.
- With this short list in hand, call the office of each pediatrician and explain that you are looking for a doctor for your baby.
- Some parents select a pediatrician based on these conversations. Others may want to interview each candidate and ask, in more detail, how the practice works.

YOU ARE NOT A BAD MOTHER IF YOU BOTTLE FEED

Q *When my baby arrives, I would like to bottle feed. But I get the feeling that I will be a terrible mother if I do. Aren't there any good things to be said about bottle feeding?*

A You will not be a bad mother if you choose to bottle feed; that's your choice. Here's a list of some of the advantages to bottle feeding that often go overlooked:

- Some women enjoy the freedom that bottle feeding provides.
- Someone else can take care of the baby.

- Fathers can be more involved in the baby's care, especially those middle-of-the-night feedings.
- Bottle fed babies typically require fewer feedings than breastfed babies.
- You can tell exactly how much formula your baby is getting at each feeding.

HELPING A CHOKING INFANT

Q *As a paramedic with 10 years' experience, I've been called several times to homes where an infant under one year of age was choking, usually on food. In most cases the child's fate was decided by the time we arrived: Someone had either relieved the blocked airway or the child had already suffered brain damage or death. Would it help to inform parents how to respond to the choking infant?*

A Good idea, especially when choking is the most common cause of accidental death in children under one year of age. Parents need to understand how to deal with these frightening situations.

Choking occurs when an object such as food "goes down the wrong way," enters the opening to the windpipe, and lodges there instead of entering the esophagus, which leads to the stomach. In response, coughing is an attempt to dislodge the object and bring it up.

To decrease the risk of choking when introducing solid foods to an infant, make sure your baby is sitting up, either in your lap or in an infant seat. Never offer an infant spoonfuls of peanut butter, pieces of raw carrot, nuts, grapes, popcorn, uncooked peas, celery, hard candies, or hot dogs.

If an infant begins coughing, gagging, or having high-pitched breathing, suspect she is choking. If she's only coughing, let her cough. Don't try to remove the object with your fingers, which could push it farther down the throat and completely block the airway.

However, if she can't breathe and is turning blue or red in the face, take emergency action. If someone is nearby, yell for them to call for assistance while you begin the following steps recommended by the American Academy of Pediatrics (AAP):

- Gently place the infant face-down on your forearm in a head down position, resting your forearm firmly against your thigh for support. Rapidly give four blows to the back, between the shoulder blades, with the heel of the hand.
- If she still can't breathe, turn her over onto her back, resting her on your thigh, and rapidly deliver four chest thrusts overthe breastbone, using only two fingers.
- If she's still not breathing, open the airway by tilting the head back until her nose is pointing toward the ceiling, and look in her mouth for the object. If you see it, remove it by sweeping the back of the mouth with your finger.
- If she's still not breathing, try giving two breaths, mouth to mouth. If you are alone with your child and she is still not breathing, repeat steps 1 to 4 as you call for emergency assistance.

A further thought: The AAP recommends that all parents and anyone else who cares for children should complete a course in the treatment for choking and CPR. You can contact your local chapter of the American Heart Association or Red Cross or your local hospital to find out where certified courses are given in your community.

RESPONDING TO A BABY'S CRY

Q *Please settle an argument between my husband and me. I say that our infant son (five weeks old) should be attended as soon as he cries, even though it means disrupting what I* *am doing to soothe him. My husband says the baby needs to learn to comfort himself, and we should let him cry as long as he's not cold, hungry, or in need of a diaper change. Who's right?*

A Your husband seems to be carrying his brand of "tough love" a bit too far. Reading between the lines, he may be worried that if he picks up his crying son and comforts him, this loving act will backfire, and he'll end up with a "spoiled" child.

Let's play pretend. Suppose you're having a particularly stressful day. At your wits end, you ask your husband to take you in his arms and just hold you. But, instead of a tender moment, he turns away.

An absurd comparison?

Perhaps.

But, remember, babies too have bad days—periods of time when their immature nervous systems get overloaded, and they blow off steam by crying. When you pick up a crying baby and just hold him, this action helps his jumpy nervous system reorganize, not unlike what happens when we give each other a hug.

Also, remember, five-week-old babies communicate by crying. One of the more difficult tasks for parents to learn is what the crying means. Does it mean he's too cold, too hot, hungry, wet, or in pain; or does it mean he longs for a tender moment with mom or dad?

We can't "spoil" a five-week-old baby (or a spouse, for that matter) by taking them in our arms and holding them. Babies and spouses only "spoil" when we turn and walk away.

You ask who's right?

Raising a child involves trying things out and learning from our mistakes. It's hard enough without keeping score.

A further thought: It's a law of nature that a crying baby will demand our attention at inconvenient times. The trick is to learn how to turn an inconvenience into an opportunity. Here's a suggestion you will hear me make repeatedly: Grab a book off the shelf and snuggle up. Use this time to read to your baby or make up your own stories. It's never too early to start.

WHY WON'T THIS THREE-MONTH-OLD STOP CRYING?

When the alarm went off, Jason's mother rolled out of bed and readied herself for work. She dressed and fed her three-month-old, loaded him in the car, then dropped him off at day care. As she drove away, Jason cooed and smiled at Miss Amy, his caretaker for the day.

Dressed in infant pajamas that enclosed his active feet, Jason loved to lie on his back and kick at the mobile hanging just above his crib. But toward noon, something unusual happened—Jason started to cry.

Miss Amy picked him up and strolled about, softly humming a tune. He seemed to settle down, but when she tried to put him down, he started up again. After awhile, nothing seemed to help.

Miss Amy thought to herself: He didn't feel warm to the touch like he would if he had a fever. He didn't pull at his ears like some babies do when they have an ear infection. Earlier, when she had changed his diaper, his bowel movement didn't look unusual. His mother hadn't mentioned that anyone was sick at home. He didn't have a runny nose or a cough. What was going on?

Finally, Miss Amy called Jason's mother at work and told her how Jason was acting. Not knowing what else to do, Jason's mother left work and drove to pick him up. On the way, she called her doctor and told him the story. He offered to see Jason as soon as she could get him there.

At the doctor's office, Jason's ears looked fine, his throat was clear, and his lungs and heart sounded fine. But when the doctor removed Jason's pajama bottom, he found the culprit: a purplish toe, double its normal size. A deep groove circled the toe at the base where it joined the foot. A loose pajama thread had wrapped around the toe and acted like a rubber band, constricting the toe and causing swelling and inflammation.

He cut the thread with a fine scissors and started antibiotics. A week later, the swelling and redness were gone.

Repeated washing of pajama bottoms produces loose threads that can wrap around a toe or even the penis, which can cause swelling and inflammation. If ignored, it can lead to gangrene and loss of the body part. A long strand of hair can also produce the same effect.

All babies cry, but excessive crying suggests something drastic is wrong. A thorough physical exam with all clothes removed will usually identify the problem.

TO WORK OR NOT TO WORK

Q *My husband and I are expecting our first child in three months. The problem is my husband wants me to quit my job and stay at home with the baby, but I'm not so sure. He manages a hardware store, and I work as a paralegal for a law firm. I love my work yet want to do what's best for the baby. Can you help us figure this out?*

A One approach couples have successfully used to resolve this important issue is to sit down with open minds and calmly discuss all options, including the possibility that either parent may stay at home with the baby. To help this process, ask yourselves the following questions and then compare answers.

- **What are my priorities?** Carefully consider the things that are most important in your life and rank order these on a piece of paper. Your list may

include your baby, your family, your career, your church, financial security, a new home, a new car, vacations, entertainment, and so on. After ranking your priorities, ask yourself whether working or staying at home will best meet the most important items on your list.
- **Which role best suits my personality?** If you stay at home, might you grow impatient or bored? If you decide to work, will you be able to leave your concerns about the baby at home? Can you compartmentalize your life so you can do your best in either case?
- **Would I feel comfortable having someone else take care of my baby?** Can you find a substitute who will take care of your baby as well as you can? Unfair question? Perhaps.
- **How much energy do I have?** It takes a lot of physical and emotional stamina to rise each morning, get ready for work, put in a full day on the job, then return to the demands of the baby, home, and spouse. If you lack energy, what often suffers most is the husband-wife relationship.
- **If I decide to work, will I get adequate support from my spouse or some other source?** Is your spouse willing to do his or her share of baby-sitting, shopping, cooking, cleaning, and laundry? Are you able to afford outside help?
- **What is our financial situation?** If you decide not to work, will it threaten your family's financial picture or just mean cutting back on extras?
- **How flexible is my job?** Is it possible to work part of the time at home? Can you take time off when your baby or the sitter becomes sick? Will you be able to arrive late or leave early if an emergency occurs at home? Does your job require long hours, weekends, or travel?

- **If I don't work, how will it affect my career?** Putting a career on hold and staying home with the baby has consequences, some good and some not so good. In your case, what might those consequences be?

Whatever choice the two of you make, please remember to find time, every day, to read to your baby.

WHAT PARENTS SHOULD KNOW ABOUT FEVER

Q *My mother says she used to sponge me down with alcohol when I was a baby and had a fever. Is it safe to use alcohol this way? How do you recommend treating a fever?*

A When it comes to treating a fever with alcohol, our thinking has changed since you were a baby. Never bathe or sponge a child with alcohol, because alcohol can be absorbed through the skin or inhaled and cause serious harm. Here are some things every parent should know about fever, including how to treat it:

- A fever is defined as an oral temperature of 100.3 degrees or higher or a rectal temperature of 101.1 degrees or higher.
- Fever itself is not a disease; it's usually a positive sign that the body is fighting an infection.
- Our body temperature varies during the day with the low point in the morning and the high point in late afternoon.
- Infected newborns may have a normal or subnormal temperature. However, they are usually irritable, lethargic, or feeding poorly if they have an illness. If your child is two months of age or younger and has a fever, call your doctor immediately.

- In children between six months and five years of age, fever can trigger seizures, called febrile convulsions. The child may look peculiar for a few moments, then stiffen up, twitch, and roll her eyes. She may be unresponsive for up to a few minutes. It's reassuring to know that febrile convulsions almost always are harmless, though they should be reported promptly to your doctor.
- A temperature under 101 degrees usually does not need to be treated unless your child is uncomfortable or has a history of febrile convulsions.
- Acetaminophen, ibuprofen, and aspirin are three medications most often used to treat a fever. All three of these drugs appear to be equally effective at reducing fever. *However, because aspirin may be associated with serious side effects, it should not be used in children.*
- In some cases of fever, you might combine medication with tepid sponging, or just sponging alone. To sponge your child, place her in one to two inches of slightly warm water. Then, using a clean wash cloth or sponge, spread a film of water over the trunk, arms and legs. The water will evaporate and cool the body. Do not use cold water; it may cause shivering and raise the body temperature.

Never leave a baby alone in water, even for an instant. If you need to answer the phone or door, you must take the baby with you.

A further thought: A rare but serious problem that is easily confused with fever is heatstroke. This condition is not caused by an infection but by excessive surrounding heat. It can occur on a hot beach in midsummer, during a hard-fought athletic event, or in an overheated, closed car. *Never leave a child unattended in a closed car, even for a few minutes.*

AVOIDING "BABY BOTTLE TOOTH DECAY"

Q *My husband and I sometimes put our four-month-old to bed with a bottle of juice. I've heard it can cause tooth decay but have never understood how. Can you explain how putting a baby to bed with a bottle causes tooth decay? Since his baby teeth are going to fall out anyway, how much does it matter if a few are decayed?*

A After falling asleep, a baby who is regularly put to bed with a bottle of milk or juice often ends up with a small pool of sugary liquid in his mouth. Once the sugar is changed to acid by bacteria in the mouth, the acid attacks the teeth and causes "baby bottle tooth decay."

If a child loses his baby teeth early because of decay, the remaining teeth may shift position to fill in the gaps, leaving no room for the permanent teeth to come in. So, it can matter a lot if baby teeth develop decay.

Here are a few more reasons to avoid putting a child to bed with a bottle of milk or juice:

- Lying on the back allows liquid to enter the middle ear through the auditory canal and cause ear infections.
- Leaving a child unattended with a bottle is potentially dangerous should he choke and need help.
- Putting a child to bed alone with a bottle deprives parents and their baby of valuable social interaction.
- Later on, parents may be in for trouble when their child refuses to give up the habit.

IS MY BABY'S TEAR DUCT BLOCKED?

Q *My two-week-old is incredibly healthy. But ever since I brought her home from the hospital, I've noticed a buildup* *of watery white matter in the corner of her right eye, especially when she wakes up from a nap. My mother says she has a blocked tear duct, the same thing I had as a baby. She thinks I should have her checked by our doctor. What do you think? Do blocked tear ducts run in families?*

A Here's why your mother is probably right. Normally, the tear ducts drain the tears through a small opening at the inner corner of each eye, emptying the tears into your baby's nasal passages. When a tear duct is blocked, the tears well up in the eye, like a stagnant pond, setting up a mild infection of the eyelids, which explains the buildup of watery white matter in the corner of your baby's eye.

Your doctor should see the eye to confirm the diagnosis. In most cases, gentle massage of the inner corner of the eye will open it up. Occasionally, an eye specialist has to open the duct with a simple procedure. As far as I know, blocked tear ducts do not run in families.

DOES MY BABY NEED A DAILY BATH?

Q *Can you please settle a slight disagreement between my mother-in-law and me? I bathe my six-week-old son every other day. She says to bathe him daily. Who is right? Is there another way?*

A Most experts suggest bathing an infant two or three times a week during the first year. If your baby is bathed more often, it may dry out his skin. Just be sure to wash the diaper area thoroughly during each diaper change.

One note of caution when giving your baby a bath: If you're called away to answer the phone or respond to a knock at the door, wrap your baby in a towel and take him with you. Never leave a baby alone in the water, even for an instant.

A further thought: Diaper pails cause numerous injuries and even deaths to young children. Naturally curious, children have even fallen headfirst into diaper pails and drowned. Always keep a diaper pail tightly closed and out of the reach of young children. When shopping for a pail, choose one with a foot-operated pedal to keep your hands free for the baby.

DO INFANTS NEED EXTRA VITAMINS?

Q *At my baby's six-week checkup, I asked her pediatrician whether I should be giving my baby vitamins. She said it wasn't necessary. What is your opinion? By the way, I feed my daughter formula containing added iron.*

A Whether bottle fed or breastfed, healthy babies receiving a normal diet do not need vitamin supplements, according to the American Academy of Pediatrics. However, some breastfed infants in urban settings who are not exposed to enough sunlight may need supplemental vitamin D.

Vitamin D is naturally manufactured by the skin when it is exposed to sunlight. All it takes is 15 minutes of sunlight a week for fair-skinned children. (Prepared formula has vitamin D added to it.) Also, babies born prematurely are usually given extra vitamins.

A further thought: Believe it or not, a first-time mother recently approached me at a social gathering and asked how to care for her baby's uncircumcised penis.

I suggested she simply clean his penis with soap and water when she gives him a bath and not try to pull his foreskin back. Why? Because the foreskin is connected by tissue to the head of the penis. Any attempt to pull it back will cause bleeding and swelling.

D. Gary Benfield, M.D.

Toward the end of the first year—after her baby's doctor indicates that the foreskin has started to separate from the penis underneath—she can begin retracting her baby's foreskin and washing the tip of his penis, remembering to always pull the foreskin forward when she is done.

MOST HEART MURMURS IN CHILDREN ARE "INNOCENT"

Q *Our 13-month-old usually passes her checkups with flying colors. But during her last visit, the doctor noticed a heart murmur, which he said not to worry about. Can you tell me what a heart murmur is? Does it mean something is wrong with her heart? I'm still concerned.*

A When you listen through a stethoscope to the sound of a child's beating heart, you may hear an additional sound called a murmur. This extra sound is usually produced by the flow of blood as it passes through the heart or the large vessels leading to and from the heart. A murmur may become more obvious following exercise or during a fever when the heart has to work harder.

Some parents mistakenly equate the presence of a heart murmur with some form of congenital heart disease. Yet studies show that 50 percent of healthy children will develop a heart murmur sometime during childhood.

In contrast, less than 1 percent of children are born with congenital heart disease, and many of them do not have a murmur. So you see, most murmurs are innocent, meaning they have no clinical significance.

On the other hand, we always consider the possibility of a heart problem when a child presents with any combination of the following, whether the child has a heart murmur or not:

- Slow feeding
- Rapid breathing

- Excessive sweating
- Slow growth or an inability to keep up with one's peers

A further thought: The worst thing a parent can do is to restrict a little child's activity when all she has is an innocent murmur. The next worst thing the parent can do is label the child as having a heart problem.

Chances are the child's self-image will suffer and adversely affect her activities among friends and later at school. When she reaches adulthood, still firmly convinced she has a heart problem, she may experience difficulty obtaining health insurance, life insurance, and certain types of employment.

Sound far-fetched?

Believe me, it's not.

WHAT IS THE APPROPRIATE ROOM TEMPERATURE FOR A BABY?

Q *Our baby is three weeks old and weighs a little over 9 pounds. Can you tell us how warm we should keep the room?*

A Most experts recommend a room temperature about 70 degrees Fahrenheit. They also suggest keeping the humidity near 50 percent. This level of humidity helps maintain the room's heat.

YOUR BABY'S SOFT SPOT IS STRONGER THAN YOU THINK

Q *Our baby has a soft spot on the top of her head. Might someone damage her brain if they accidentally press on it?*

A That type of injury is unlikely to happen, because the soft spot you are referring to is covered by strong, fibrous tissue. It usually closes between 12 and 18 months of age when the skull bones finish growing together.

TAKING YOUR BABY'S TEMPERATURE

Q *So far, I haven't had to take my two-week-old baby's temperature, but, when I do, I'm afraid I might do something wrong and either harm my baby or get an incorrect reading. Can you explain how to take a baby's temperature?*

A Let's start with a digital thermometer, which you can buy at a drugstore for less than $10.

Here's how to take your baby's temperature rectally, the preferred way at least until your baby is three months old:

- Wash the end with soap and water and rinse it with running water.
- Rub a small amount of petroleum jelly on the end.
- Lay your baby face down across your lap or on a firm surface.
- Press the thermometer button to turn it on.
- Gently spread your baby's buttocks apart with one hand, and then insert the lubricated end approximately one inch into the rectum using your other hand.
- When the thermometer beeps, remove it and read your baby's temperature.

Call your doctor if your baby is under three months old and has a rectal temperature higher than 100.4 degrees or if your baby has an increase in temperature along with symptoms such as difficulty breathing, listlessness, diarrhea, or vomiting.

A further thought: Never give aspirin to lower your child's fever. The use of aspirin has been linked to an increased risk of Reyes' syndrome, a rare but serious disease that affects the brain and liver.

BRUSHING UP ON HEALTHY TEETH

Q *I want my daughter to have pretty teeth and a nice smile when she grows up. Her first tooth is just starting to come in. Can you tell me how and when I should start cleaning her teeth? We have county water that contains fluoride. Is that enough for healthy teeth or will I need to use extra fluoride later on?*

A As soon as the first tooth appears, clean the tooth daily by wiping it with a clean, damp cloth. When more teeth come in, switch to a small, soft toothbrush, using a dab of toothpaste. Most young children do not enjoy having their teeth brushed, so try sitting your daughter sideways on your knee. Hold her with one arm, and use the other to brush.

Parents should brush their child's teeth until the child can handle the toothbrush alone. Children usually develop this skill around the age of four or five.

You will hear all kinds of advice on whether the best brushing motion is up or down, back and forth, or around in circles. The truth is the direction really doesn't matter, according to most dentists.

What's important is to clean each tooth thoroughly, top and bottom, inside and out. Here you may encounter resistance from your child, who probably will concentrate on only the front teeth she can see. It may help to turn it into a game of "find the hidden teeth."

Babies do not require extra fluoride during the first six months of life, according to the American Academy of Pediatrics. After that, if your water contains less than .3 parts per million of fluoride, your daughter may need extra fluoride. Check with your doctor to find out if fluoride drops are necessary in the area where you live.

Further thoughts:

- To help prevent cavities, never let your baby fall asleep with a bottle of milk or carbohydrate-containing liquid, either at nap time or at night. In this way, you will keep the liquid from pooling around the teeth and creating a breeding ground for decay.
- All 20 baby teeth, or primary teeth, begin forming in the jaw bones before a baby is born. The two lower central front teeth are usually the first to come through, followed by the upper two. All four usually appear between six months and one year of age. All 20 primary teeth usually come in by 24 to 30 months of age.
- The first of the 32 permanent teeth usually start to come in around the age of six. A full set of permanent teeth is usually in between 17 and 20 years of age.
- Most dentists suggest parents make the first appointment when all 20 primary teeth are in, sometime between 24 and 30 months of age. During this visit, your dentist will examine your child's teeth to make sure they are coming in normally, check for any dental problems, and teach the two of you the basics of good dental care.

Grandparenting

UNDERSTANDING YOUR NEW GRANDCHILD

Q *I'll never forget that special moment when my first grandchild was born. After his parents took turns holding him, my* *daughter handed him to me. As if on cue, he opened his eyes and gazed straight into mine. When I whispered over and over how much we loved him, his eyes followed mine as if we were having a conversation. Was his response unusual or do babies normally respond this way right after they are born?*

A Scientists have shown that newborn behavior is organized into six different states of consciousness:

- Two sleep states: quiet sleep and active sleep
- Three awake states: quiet alert, active alert, and crying
- Drowsiness: a transition state between sleep and wakefulness

You observed one of the newborn's first responses after birth, the tendency to move into a *quiet alert state* of consciousness. While in this state, which may last up to 40 minutes, a baby will follow a red ball, imitate his holder's facial movements, and respond to voices.

All of his energy seems to be focused on seeing, hearing, and responding. Most babies spend about 10 percent of each day in this receptive state, searching to understand the world.

During the *active alert state,* a baby makes frequent movements and small sounds, and looks about the room. This state often signals when a baby is hungry.

Babies enter a *drowsy state* when they are waking up or falling asleep. Their eyes take on a dull, glazed appearance and usually do not focus.

During the newborn period, infants sleep about 90 percent of the time, alternating in 30 minute intervals between quiet and active sleep. In the *active sleep state,* an infant's eyes are usually closed, but occasionally they will flutter from closed to open. The term *rapid eye movement*

(REM) sleep comes from the eye movements during this type of restless sleep.

Infants in this state often make funny faces—grimaces, smiles, frowns—and may display chewing movements or bursts of sucking. Adults experience REM sleep when they are dreaming; we aren't totally sure whether the same is true for newborns.

In the *crying state,* babies often communicate discomfort or hunger. However, parents who pick up their crying babies and hold them against their shoulder are giving them a chance to quiet down and learn about the world by scanning the room.

A further thought: Parents and grandparents alike can learn a lot by closely observing their children and grandchildren. It all begins at birth. Unfortunately, all too often, we adults are so busy and self-absorbed that we dull our powers of observation, lose patience with our children, and no longer trust ourselves to figure out what they are really trying to tell us.

FIRST-TIME GRANDMOTHER

Q *I'll soon be a first-time grandmother. Can you suggest how to walk the line between helping my daughter after the baby arrives and not getting in her way?*

A You can start off by offering to be there for your daughter after the baby is born, to help get meals and help out around the house, but be wary about offering unsolicited advice. Learning to parent means learning from mistakes. And parents must make them for themselves. If you are ready to listen and, if asked, to help her sort out her mistakes, both of you may become better parents.

CHILDREN OF LESBIAN, GAY PARENTS

Q *I am a somewhat unusual grandparent. My daughter and her lesbian partner have a beautiful six-week-old baby. She was conceived in my daughter's body using artificial insemination. I usually support my daughter's choices, but I'm concerned about my granddaughter's future. Can you tell me whether it's safe for the baby to be raised in that environment? Is she more likely to grow up a lesbian?*

A Other grandparents have voiced similar concerns about their lesbian or gay children having and raising children. They worry about a number of things:

- Their grandchildren will grow up lesbian or gay.
- They will be psychologically damaged and have more behavior problems than children raised in traditional heterosexual families.
- They will be teased and stigmatized by their peers.
- They will be sexually or physically abused by their parents or by their parents' friends.

Here is what some of the latest research says about these issues:

- In general, children of lesbian or gay parents do not seem to function differently from children in traditional families.
- No differences were found in adolescent sexual orientation, the frequency of psychiatric difficulties, personality characteristics, moral maturity, or intelligence.
- Although children of lesbian mothers reported greater stress, they also reported a greater sense of well-being than children growing up in heterosexual families.

D. Gary Benfield, M.D.

- Children of lesbian parents tend to be less aggressive than their peers and more affectionate and protective toward younger children.
- Children of lesbian and gay parents are less likely to be sexually or physically abused by their parents or their parents' friends, contrary to what some people might think.

In the past, most children of lesbians and gay men were conceived before their lesbian and gay parents recognized or admitted their sexual orientation. More recently, however, growing numbers of lesbians and gay men are becoming parents by adopting or foster parenting. Like your daughter, lesbians may also become parents by using artificial insemination. Gay men may father children through arrangements with friends or surrogates.

We are going to see more written about the emergence of lesbian and gay families. How grandparents fit in is only one of the many unanswered questions. Stay tuned.

A further thought: About 77 percent of white children, 67 percent of Hispanic children, and 37 percent of black children currently live with both biological parents, according to the Census Bureau. A quarter of all U.S. children live in single-parent households, 22 percent with their mothers, and 3 percent with their fathers. In contrast, in 1970, 12 percent of all U.S. children lived with one parent—11 percent with their mothers and 1 percent with their fathers.

CAN'T DOCTORS AND NURSES SPEAK ENGLISH?

Q *As parents of three grown children and grandparents of four more, my husband and I thought we knew something about babies until our fifth grandchild was born premature.*

Walking the Baby Beat

When we visited the baby on the neonatal ward, the doctors and nurses were friendly but very hard to understand. One doctor said the baby's lytes were out of whack, and they were going to adjust the TPN to get back in the middle of the road. It sounded more like he was fixing a car than a sick baby. A nurse said since the baby was LGA, he might be an IDM. These abbreviations drove us crazy. Can you explain what they mean? By the way, you don't talk that way, do you?

A I couldn't help but smile at your story. I must admit, sometimes I do talk that way. Like other specialties in pediatrics, neonatology has its own language and alphabet-soup shorthand.

- The baby's "lytes" stands for *serum electrolytes,* the level of sodium, potassium, and chloride—important minerals for cellular function—in the baby's blood.
- *TPN* or *total parenteral nutrition* refers to an intravenous solution containing protein, fat, sugar, vitamins, minerals, and water.
- *LGA* means *large for gestational age.*
- *IDM* stands for *infant of a diabetic mother.*

These and a myriad of other terms often become part of a parent's everyday conversation while her baby is in intensive care. Seriously, I trust your grandson is now fully recovered and doing well at home.

A further thought: Here's a list of the "Top 10 Foods That Cause Choking" in children under four:

Apples	Carrots
Celery	Nuts
Grapes	Peanut butter
Hard candy	Popcorn
Hot dogs	Raisins

D. Gary Benfield, M.D.

GRANDPARENTS CAN MAKE A DIFFERENCE

Q *Our first grandchild, Emily Ann, was born almost three weeks ago. Her mother (also our daughter), Susan, was bleeding and had to have an emergency cesarean 14 weeks before she was supposed to deliver. Emily Ann weighed a few ounces less than two pounds and has been in intensive care all this time.*

The doctors have weaned her from the breathing machine, she no longer needs extra oxygen, and they're feeding her breast milk through a tube that goes in her nose down to her stomach. The doctors say she is doing beautifully. They say she hasn't had any brain bleeds or any other bad complications.

They've got Susan so excited that she fully expects Emily Ann to survive and be healthy. Isn't it a bit early to be so optimistic? Won't it take years before we really know whether she's okay? I'm concerned that Susan will get her hopes up and something will still go wrong, sooner or later. I don't mean to be a wet blanket, just concerned.

A At times like this, grandparents walk a fine line. On one hand, you want to be supportive, optimistic, and upbeat. You may show your support by helping your daughter with her daily chores and fixing meals, freeing her up to be with Emily Ann as much as possible. On the other hand, you have concerns. You may even know of another family who had a similar experience to what your daughter is going through, and things didn't turn out so well. Here are a few thoughts to help you walk that line:

- If Emily Ann was born 14 weeks early, that means she was born at 26 weeks gestation since full term is 40 weeks.
- From your description, it sounds like your granddaughter has done as well as anyone could hope for, especially for a baby born this early.

Walking the Baby Beat

- She no longer needs help with her breathing, does not need extra oxygen, is taking tube feedings, and hasn't suffered any complications so far.
- Though she's not completely out of the woods, her chances for survival from the moment she was born were better than 9 out of 10. Now that she's gotten this far without complications, her chances are even better than that.
- We all know that survival is one thing, being completely healthy is another. And yes, it will take some time to know for sure whether she's completely healthy.
- But when you think about it, that's true of all newborns, those born early or those born on time. There's always uncertainty about each baby's future health.

So, as a grandparent, if I'm going to err as I walk that line, I prefer to err on the side of optimism rather than pessimism.

Why? Because pessimism is just as contagious as optimism. If your concerns spill over onto your daughter, she may hold back, not daring to fully bond with Emily Ann for fear that if something goes wrong it will hurt even more.

I know that sounds irrational and even a bit uncaring, but we see examples of this hesitation in the neonatal intensive care unit all the time.

For instance, the couple who holds off for days giving their critically ill baby a name for fear that if the baby dies it will hurt even more. Or the couple who can't bring themselves to visit their seriously ill baby because they may become too attached.

Irrational? Yes. But it makes sense to those parents at the time.

So if I were you, I'd help out as best I can and be optimistically involved in little Emily Ann's future. You too can make a difference in how she turns out.

Immunizations

CHILD'S COLD NOT A GOOD REASON TO POSTPONE SHOTS

Q *Our nine-month-old has a doctor's appointment for his shots, but he has a runny nose and a slight fever. Should I keep the appointment or reschedule?*

A An acute infection—with or without a low-grade fever—is not an indication to postpone a child's immunizations. You might call your doctor to make sure this agrees with his office policy.

A further thought: Some parents have the mistaken impression that if a child misses an immunization, he will have to restart the whole series to catch up. Immunizations should resume from the point of interruption, regardless of how much time has passed since the last dose.

ARE ALL THOSE SHOTS REALLY NECESSARY?

Q *When we took our baby home from the hospital, the nurse gave us a schedule of baby shots. For the first year he'll be getting a shot just about every time he sees the doctor. Can you tell me why so many shots? Are they all really necessary?*

A Those "baby shots" contain vaccines to protect your child against 10 childhood diseases: polio, measles, mumps, rubella (German measles), pertussis (whooping cough), diphtheria, tetanus, haemophilus infections, hepatitis, and varicella (chickenpox). Those diseases can cause serious illness and even death.

Take the Hib vaccine, for example. It's a vaccine that prevents infections caused by Haemophilus influenzae type b or H. flu for short. Before the vaccine was developed, H. flu caused about 12,000 cases of meningitis each year in children younger than five.

Of those 12,000 children, one in 20 died and one in four suffered permanent brain damage. H. flu also causes epiglottitis, a dangerous infection of the throat; pneumonia; and serious infections involving the blood, bones, joints, skin, and heart. Without protection of the Hib vaccine, your baby could suffer from this serious but preventable disease.

In case you're still not convinced, let's look back in history at two other preventable diseases: whooping cough and polio. In 1916, whooping cough killed more than 10,000 children in the United States. That same year an epidemic of more than 29,000 cases of polio struck the East Coast, causing more than 6,000 deaths. Of the children who survived that epidemic, many were crippled for life.

A lot of shots? Yes.

Are they really necessary? You bet!

IS IT IMPORTANT TO IMMUNIZE YOUR CHILD AGAINST CHICKENPOX?

Q *My baby's immunization schedule says she'll need a shot of Varivax to prevent chickenpox at 12 months of age. Can you tell me why it was added to what seems like an already overcrowded list of immunizations? Does my child really need another shot? Is it safe?*

A Once upon a time, the rash of chickenpox (varicella) was looked upon as something all kids got. (I still remember my mom warning me not to scratch the itchy "spots" as she dabbed them with cotton balls soaked in Calamine lotion. "If you scratch the scab off, you will be scarred for life," she said.)

For most of us, the infection was nothing more than an annoying, itchy rash. And because it was so common, families and most doctors were unaware of how serious it could be for some children and adults.

In fact, chickenpox was never just an annoying, trivial disease. Consider these statistics, before the chickenpox vaccine was introduced in 1995:

- Four million cases annually, 90 percent of them in children
- Eleven thousand hospitalizations, 60 percent of them in children
- One hundred and five deaths, 45 percent of them in children
- Substantial medical and societal costs

For these reasons, a chickenpox vaccine was added to the list of immunizations children now receive, and explains why many states require that a child be vaccinated against chickenpox before entering day care or school.

What complications of chickenpox caused all those hospitalizations and deaths? Bacterial infection of the skin and difficulty with blood clotting that resulted in bleeding under the skin and internal hemorrhage were the two most common complications.

Other complications included arthritis, hepatitis, encephalitis, meningitis, and inflammation of the kidneys. Reye's syndrome—when aspirin was commonly used to reduce fever—also caused liver failure and death.

The incidence of these complications has been greatly reduced since the chickenpox vaccine has become widely used.

Is the vaccine safe? More than 40 million doses of the vaccine have been given, and severe side effects have been extremely rare. The risk of complications from chickenpox is far greater than the risk of complications from the vaccine.

When should a child be vaccinated? One dose of the vaccine is recommended for children 12 to 18 months of age who have not had chickenpox. Children who don't get the vaccine then can get it at any age. Those older than 13 should get two doses, four to eight weeks apart.

Further thoughts: The vaccine is also recommended if an unimmunized child or adult is exposed to someone with the disease. The vaccine shows good protection if it's given within three days of exposure.

Can you get chickenpox after being vaccinated? No vaccine is 100 percent effective. So the answer is "Yes."

Chickenpox in a child who has been vaccinated is called "breakthrough" disease. Breakthrough chickenpox is mild: less than 50 spots, compared to the 300 to 500 spots typical of regular chickenpox and a brief illness lasting two or three days.

What if a susceptible pregnant woman comes into contact with chickenpox? The vaccine cannot be given in pregnancy, but she should still inform her doctor right away about the exposure. She may benefit from an injection of immune globulin to modify the disease.

ROUTINE SMALLPOX VACCINATION NO LONGER AVAILABLE

Q *I was vaccinated against smallpox back in the early 1970s. Can you tell me whether I have lifelong immunity? If not, should I get vaccinated again?*

A Vaccination against smallpox does not confer lifelong immunity. Routine vaccination for smallpox stopped in the United States in 1980, so immunity acquired before that time has waned. Therefore, previously vaccinated persons are considered susceptible to smallpox, along with everyone else.

The Centers for Disease Control and Prevention (CDC) oversees the only remaining supply of smallpox vaccine in this country, which is not available to you or me. So you can't get vaccinated again for smallpox even if you want to.

A further thought: The federal government announced a controversial decision to use the remaining stock of American smallpox samples to develop several antiviral drugs and a vaccine that can be used to immunize the whole country.

Perhaps the time will come when we are once again required to be vaccinated for smallpox.

Toddler time

OUR TODDLER IS DRIVING US NUTS!

Q *Our 17-month-old daughter is driving us nuts! Whether the issue is getting dressed, going to bed, or taking a bath, she delights in saying "No." How should we handle her behavior? Can you give us some idea how long it will last?*

A All children, more or less, go through this negative phase in search of independence and a new identity. So don't take it personally. By "No" she probably means, "Do I have to?" or "Do you mean it?" She doesn't mean to annoy you. Try to look at it with a sense of humor. Here are several suggestions:

- Give your daughter choices. In this way, you increase her sense of freedom and control so she will become more cooperative. Let her choose which toys to take in the tub, which book to read, and which breakfast cereal to eat.
- Don't give her a choice when none exists. Whether to sit in the car seat is not open to debate: Safety rules. However, you can explain why she must follow the rule. Going to bed is another example.
- Allow transition time when changing activities. If your child is having fun, give her a five-minute warning as dinnertime approaches.

Should you punish her for saying "No"? When necessary, discipline your child for what she does, not what she says. If you argue about saying "No," you will probably prolong the behavior. On average, this phase of development lasts about a year.

A further thought: Parents should read to and play with their toddler every day. Choose books that encourage touching and pointing to objects. Get down on the floor with your child and have fun.

WHEN TODDLERS DISCOVER THEIR GENITALS

Q *My husband and I disagree about a problem with our twins and would like your help. But before we get to the problem, let me tell you about us.*

I'm 40 years old, a lawyer, and an only child. My father's a retired Baptist minister who was very strict about dating and drinking and, well, you can guess the rest.

On the other hand, my husband, who's also a 40-year-old lawyer, is the oldest of five children. His parents both worked, so he was heavily involved in helping raise his younger siblings. His parents were more laid back and less strict than mine.

D. Gary Benfield, M.D.

Now, to our problem: Our 25-month-old twins, a boy and a girl, are normal, healthy kids in every way except for one thing: they have both started to play with their genitals, but, thankfully, not with each other's. I usually react by smacking their hands and telling them to stop. When my husband's around, he gives me an icy stare, but says nothing.

We have talked about it in private; he takes the kids' side, claiming I'm overreacting. He says if we just leave them alone, they'll stop, sooner or later. What do you think?

A I consulted three different sources—The American Academy of Pediatrics, *Dr. Spock's Baby and Child Care* book, and William and Martha Sears' *The Baby Book*—for advice about your concern. All three basically agree on the reasons why toddlers often play with their genitals and how parents should respond.

It's normal for a toddler to explore various body parts. This exploration usually involves thumb sucking and finger play in the first year, and progresses to penis pulling and vaginal probing during the second year.

At some point, natural curiosity leads to the pleasure of self-stimulation. Like thumb sucking, the ability to stimulate body parts for pleasure is a normal part of growing up. And even if this behavior induces a penile erection in boys, it's neither a sexual nor emotional experience for toddlers. It just feels good.

If you show a strong negative reaction when your twins touch their genitals, you're suggesting that something is wrong or bad about these body parts and that something's wrong with your twins.

Try not to discourage it, worry about it, or call attention to it. Wait until they're older to teach them about privacy and modesty. For now, try to relax and accept their behavior as normal curiosity.

By the way, here's advanced warning for when your twins turn three. Around that age, boys and girls become openly interested in each other's bodies. It's called "show and touch." Other names include "playing house" and "doctor and nurse."

A further thought: Some parents believe that genital stimulation may lead to that habit called masturbation. However, modern research suggests these facts:

- Masturbation is not a naughty, nasty, dirty habit.
- Masturbation does not cause insanity, mental retardation, physical deformities, blindness, pimples, hair on the palm of your hand, epilepsy, sterility, homosexuality, or sexual perversion.
- Those parents who threaten a child with these myths won't stop the child from masturbating, but they may cause the child to masturbate with lots of guilt and anxiety.
- And, when none of the threats come true, children may doubt other things their parents tell them about sex.

TIRED TODDLER'S SELF-COMFORTING HABIT

Q *When he's tired, our two-and-a-half year old sucks his thumb and jams his hand into his diaper and holds his penis. Is this normal behavior? Should we be concerned?*

A Sucking his thumb and holding his penis are usually comforting behaviors for a tired toddler your son's age. He will eventually stop, sooner if you ignore him.

HOW MUCH TV SHOULD A TODDLER WATCH?

Q *I work three 12-hour shifts a week as a nurse in a coronary care unit. While I'm working, an elderly woman whom*

D. Gary Benfield, M.D.

we trust and like very much stays with our 18-month-old daughter until my husband gets home from work. Our sitter and daughter spend much of the day watching childrens' shows and the soaps on TV. Is it harmful for a child this age to watch so much TV? Can you offer any suggestions?

A Children under the age of two should not watch television period, according to the American Academy of Pediatrics. In a recently published policy statement, the AAP cites a growing body of research on early brain development to support its position.

These studies show that babies and toddlers need to directly interact with parents and other caregivers for healthy brain growth and the development of social, emotional, and cognitive skills. To sit and watch television for hours on end deprives the brain of important chances to participate actively in creative play. It may have deleterious and irreversible consequences for the growing brain in several different ways including the following:

- Higher levels of television viewing correlate with lower academic performance, especially reading scores, perhaps because a young brain manipulated by jazzy visual effects cannot divide attention to listen carefully to language. Moreover, the "two-minute-mind" easily becomes impatient with any reading material that requires time to process.
- The fast-paced, attention-grabbing way that children's programming is presented is modeled after advertising research, which has shown that this technique is the best way to engage the brain's attention involuntarily. Such exposure deprives the child of practice in using his own brain independently, as in games, hobbies, and social interaction. This may predispose some children to attention problems.

- "Mindless" television or video games may idle and even block the development of that part of the brain responsible for self-control, moral judgment, and attention. Until we know more about the effects of TV on brain development, it seems a grave error to expose young children to a stimulus that may adversely affect this area of the brain.

What can parents do about this important issue? If you have access to the Internet, bookmark the "You and Your Family" section on the AAP's Web site (www.AAP.org) and visit it frequently. Read over their "Smart Guide to Kid's TV." It will teach you how to build a balanced TV diet for your family.

A further thought: Currently, the average American child or adolescent spends more than 21 hours per week passively viewing television. This chunk of time often displaces involvement in creative, active, or social pursuits.

WHEN A TODDLER HAS BAD BREATH

Q *My 19-month-old has bad breath even though I help her brush her teeth twice a day. Can you tell me whether her bad breath is normal?*

A Compared to adults, it's unusual for young children to have bad breath. Usually, regular brushing solves the problem. Because lack of brushing is not the reason, let's consider other possible causes.

Not surprisingly, toddlers have a knack for inserting foreign objects up their nose. In fact, it is one of the more common causes of prolonged bad breath. When a foreign body is the culprit, a parent will usually notice a discharge oozing, off and on, from the nose. Your doctor can remove it using special forceps.

Other causes of bad breath include an infection of the mouth, a sore throat, tonsillitis, or a sinus infection. A severely decaying tooth can also lead to bad breath.

A trip to the doctor seems indicated to rule out these possibilities.

IS THIS TODDLER'S HEART BEATING TOO FAST?

Q *Our 18-month-old daughter has always been a happy and healthy child. But when I took her in for a checkup recently, the doctor said her heart was beating 120 times each minute. He said that is too fast and referred us to a cardiologist.*

We have an appointment in two weeks. Can you tell me what the normal heart rate is for a child this age? I'm worried sick.

A From birth to one year of age, the heart normally beats 140 times per minute. From one to four years of age, it beats about 120 times per minute. From four to 12, it beats 100 beats per minute. After 12, it's 80 beats per minute, close to most adults. As you see, your daughter's heart rate falls within the normal range for her age.

Perhaps her doctor had another reason to refer you to a cardiologist, but just didn't explain it well or you didn't hear it. I suggest you talk with her doctor and ask again why he referred her to a cardiologist. If it turns out that her heart rate is the only reason, then you may be all worked up over a normal finding.

TODDLERS GET APPENDICITIS TOO

Q *Recently, my 20-month-old son's appendix ruptured, and he got peritonitis. The little guy almost died but was saved by* *intravenous antibiotics. What can you tell me about appendicitis in children this age? Is it true that appendicitis occurs more often in boys?*

A Acute appendicitis is the most common condition requiring emergency abdominal surgery in childhood. In the United States, almost 2 percent of children treated for appendicitis are under two years of age. Among the 80,000 cases of appendicitis that occur annually in children, 2 percent represents about 1,600 cases, which is still a sizeable number.

Appendicitis is difficult to diagnose in toddlers, which probably explains why appendicitis leads to perforation in three out of four children in the one- to four-year-old age group. Here's why:

- Oftentimes, the child shows no fever.
- Vomiting doesn't always occur, but a loss of appetite is common.
- Typically, pain occurs around the navel for several hours before it shifts to the lower right side.

The danger is that the inflamed appendix will burst and spread infection throughout the abdomen. This condition is known as peritonitis.

Appendicitis can reach the point of rupturing in less than 24 hours; therefore, any stomachache that persists for more than an hour or two should be discussed with your doctor.

The majority of cases of appendicitis do occur in boys.

Infectious diseases

WHAT'S THE DIFFERENCE BETWEEN A COLD AND THE FLU?

Q *Can you explain the difference between a common cold and the flu? Is a vaccine available for both or just the flu?*

D. Gary Benfield, M.D.

A Let's first review what a common cold and influenza (the flu) have in common, then talk about how they differ.

What a common cold and the flu have in common:

- Both diseases are highly contagious, and both are caused by viruses that attack the nose and throat. Because they are caused by viruses, antibiotics don't work to cure them.
- Both diseases are spread directly when an infected person coughs, sneezes, or speaks, sending the virus into the air for others to inhale. The virus then enters the nose and throat and begins to multiply.
- Both viruses are also spread indirectly when an infected person touches her nose or coughs and sneezes onto her hand and touches another person.
- The basic treatment for both diseases is also similar. Infected children should get extra rest, drink lots of liquids, and take medicines that *do not* contain aspirin to help bring down a fever and relieve symptoms. Children's acetaminophen or ibuprofen can be used for this purpose.
- Washing the hands after covering the face when coughing or sneezing helps prevent the spread of both diseases. Decongestants, antihistamines, and expectorants should be used only with the advice of a child's doctor.

How a common cold and the flu differ:

- Influenza differs from a common cold in several important ways. In this country, the flu is typically caused by two different influenza viruses: types A and B. Both of these types have different strains,

and the type and strain of flu virus that causes most cases varies each year. That's why individuals at risk for a serious influenza infection should receive a flu shot annually.
- The flu usually comes on suddenly and may include these "flu-like" symptoms:
  - Extreme tiredness or fatigue
  - Muscle aches and pains
  - Fever, chills, and shaking
  - A dry, hacking cough
  - A sore throat and nasal congestion
- Most children and adults who get the flu recover in one to two weeks. However, about 20,000 people in the United States die each year from the flu and its complications.
- Those who get the flu are at greatest risk for life-threatening complications include the elderly, anyone with a chronic medical condition, and young children.
- A yearly flu shot is recommended by the Centers for Disease Control and Prevention (CDC) for the following high-risk groups:
  - Adults and children, six months of age and older, who have chronic heart or lung conditions, including asthma
  - Adults and children, six months of age and older, who need regular medical care for diabetes, chronic kidney disease, or a weakened immune system
  - Children and teenagers who are on long-term aspirin therapy
  - Women who will be more than three months pregnant during the flu season
  - Residents of nursing homes and other long-term care facilities
  - All persons aged 50 years and older

In comparison to influenza, the common cold is caused by many different viruses, making it is impossible to develop an effective vaccine.

The typical symptoms of a common cold include sore throat; runny nose and watery eyes; sneezing; slight fever; decreased appetite; and a cough.

Most children will average eight to ten colds during the first two years of life. Fortunately, most colds go away by themselves and do not lead to anything worse.

However, if a child three months of age or younger develops signs of a cold, parents should always call their doctor. A cold in a youngster this age can quickly turn into a more serious illness such as bronchiolitis, croup, or pneumonia.

A further thought: The flu season usually starts in November and lasts through April. Children at risk for a serious influenza infection—six months of age and older—as well as their household contacts, should get their flu shots before the season starts.

OVERUSE OF ANTIBIOTICS CAN BE HARMFUL

Q *Recently, our four-month-old daughter was sent home from day care with a runny nose and a cough. The next day, I stayed home from work and took her to our doctor. He said she had a cold virus that was going around the community. When I asked for an antibiotic, he said she didn't need one. Wouldn't an antibiotic have cleared her up sooner and saved me from missing five days of work?*

A When a child is new to their practice, many doctors will set aside a few minutes to explain their approach to prescribing antibiotics for childhood infections. Then parents won't expect an antibiotic every time their child comes down with a cold. If your daughter had a cold, an antibiotic would not have cleared her up sooner and could have caused harm. Here's why:

- Two types of germs—bacteria and viruses—cause most infections. Viral infections are not affected by antibiotics, whereas bacterial infections are.
- All colds and most cases of bronchitis and upper respiratory infections are caused by viruses. Our job as doctors and as parents is to do the best we can to keep these children comfortable until the illness has run its course. For working parents, that may mean staying home from work.
- The overuse of antibiotics induces new strains of antibiotic-resistant bacteria to appear in the population. This resistance is rapidly becoming a major problem in this country, especially in the hospital setting and in many communities.
- The only way to treat these resistant bacteria is to admit the child to the hospital and try more powerful antibiotics which are given through the vein. In a four-month-old, this can turn into a life-threatening situation.

Unfortunately, not all doctors are as cautious as your doctor seems to be. For instance, here are the results of a survey of the way a sample of doctors prescribe antibiotics for children:

- Antibiotics were prescribed for 44 percent of children with common colds.
- Antibiotics were prescribed for 46 percent with upper respiratory infections.
- Antibiotics were prescribed for 75 percent with bronchitis.

Note: These conditions typically do not respond to antibiotics.

The reasons doctors seemed to overuse antibiotics varied as follows:

- Some were so busy that writing an antibiotic prescription was perceived as more time-efficient than explaining to parents why one was not needed.
- Some gave in to parent pressure—against their better judgment—to keep parents satisfied.
- Some doctors still didn't seem to know any better.

Sometimes a viral infection can lead to a secondary bacterial infection. Prescribing antibiotics in advance, to prevent the possibility of an eventual bacterial infection, doesn't work.

It's important to let your doctor know if a viral illness gets worse or lasts longer than expected. Then the treatment can be adjusted, as needed.

A further thought: Most youngsters will come down with eight to ten colds before they reach the age of two. If a child is in day care, or if there are older, school-age children at home, parents can expect even more infections because colds spread easily among children in close contact with each other.

HOW DOES SWIMMER'S EAR DIFFER FROM OTITIS MEDIA?

Q *Our five-year-old swims year round. He recently had an earache, so I made an appointment and took him to see his pediatrician. The doctor diagnosed swimmer's ear and put him on ear drops three times a day for a week and no swimming* *for a week. We followed the plan, and the earache cleared up beautifully. But I'm confused. Can you please tell me what actually causes swimmer's ear? How does swimmer's ear differ from a regular ear infection?*

A Let me explain some things about the ear before answering your questions.

The ear is divided into three parts: the outer ear, the middle ear, and the inner ear. The outer ear includes the ear lobe and the ear canal. The outer ear gathers sound waves traveling through the air and channels them inward through the ear canal. When sound waves reach the eardrum, they make the eardrum vibrate.

The middle ear includes the eardrum and three tiny bones: hammer, anvil, and stirrup. These three bones pick up the vibrations from the eardrum and send them to the inner ear, deep within the bones of the skull.

The vibrations stimulate nerve endings in the inner ear, which then send sound messages to the brain.

One other important part of the middle ear is the Eustachian tube, a hollow tube that runs from the middle ear to the back of the nose and throat. Its main function is to equalize the pressure on both sides of the ear drum, which helps prevent fluid buildup behind the eardrum.

Now, back to your questions. Swimmer's ear is an infection of the lining of the ear canal. Also called external otitis, swimmer's ear typically doesn't involve the ear drum.

Swimmer's ear often occurs after swimming or other activities that allow water to enter the ear canals. Swimmer's ear develops because moisture in the ear canal encourages the growth of bacteria, causing the lining of the ear canal to soften, and allows bacteria to invade the moistened lining and grow there.

Any injury to the ear canal—especially from using Q-Tips to clean the ear canal—can also allow bacteria to invade the lining of the ear canal and cause otitis externa.

D. Gary Benfield, M.D.

A regular ear infection—also known as otitis media—is an infection of the middle ear. Swimmer's ear and otitis media can both cause earache and fever. Typically, however, otitis media is often associated with having a cold while swimmer's ear is not.

To make the correct diagnosis, a doctor must examine the ears using a lighted instrument called an otoscope. With swimmer's ear, the ear canal looks reddened, swollen, and clogged with debris that may drain from the ear. On the other hand, with a middle ear infection, the ear canal is usually clear, but the eardrum looks reddened and bulges outward from fluid buildup behind the eardrum.

Repeated middle ear infections can lead to permanent hearing loss. So it's important to follow the prescribed treatment, which may or may not include antibiotics, and to keep all follow-up appointments. Swimmer's ear may cause temporary hearing loss from the swollen and partially blocked ear canal. Cleaning out the ear canal—which should only be done by a doctor—and following the prescribed treatment, as you did, clears up any temporary hearing loss.

A further thought: Before prescribing antibiotics for children, the doctor usually asks if the child has any drug allergies. In this situation parents often mention their own drug allergies, thinking that their child may have a similar reaction to these drugs.

Though this rarely happens, two recent experiences taught Howard Bennett, M.D., a pediatrician in Bethesda, Maryland, the importance of paying attention to parents' allergy history for the *parent's sake.*

In both cases, Bennett put a child on liquid Amoxicillin knowing the mother's history of penicillin allergy. Unfortunately, both mothers licked their fingers after giving the Amoxicillin to their children.

One mother immediately developed an itchy rash that responded to oral Benadryl; the other mother's reaction was more severe, requiring a trip to the emergency room. She responded to intravenous epinephrine and antihistamines without complications.

So, for all you mothers and fathers who are allergic to penicillin or other drugs, never lick your fingers after giving your child an oral dose of any drug that you are allergic to; wash your hands instead.

ARE PET IGUANAS SAFE FOR CHILDREN?

Q *Our five-year-old son just loves to go next door and visit our neighbor's pet iguana. Now he wants one for his birthday. My husband seems to support the idea, but I'm not so sure. I'm especially concerned about our six-month-old being around that kind of pet. Just how safe are these animals? Is this a good idea?*

A Apparently your son has caught "Reptile Rage," the wave of excitement sweeping the country over owning a pet reptile. Statistics show that approximately 3 percent of American households now own more than 7 million reptiles.

But what many animal lovers don't know is that these pets carry salmonella bacteria that can cause life-threatening illness, especially in children. Even in homes where young children are not permitted to touch or come in contact with the animals, they may still become infected, according to a study published in the *Journal of Pediatrics.*

Like most reptiles, iguanas carry salmonella in their intestinal tracts. The bacteria are shed periodically in the animals' feces, and that's how the bacteria gets on the animals' skin, their cages, and other materials they touch. When humans touch the animals or their cages then pick up food and eat it or put their fingers to their mouths, the bacteria are swallowed and invade our intestinal tracts.

Salmonella infection is not a disease to be taken lightly:

- A six-week-old boy in Ohio was hospitalized with diarrhea, stiff neck, and fever. He was treated and released from the hospital after 56 days.
- Vomiting, bloody diarrhea, and fever put a three-week-old Pennsylvania girl in the hospital. She was treated with penicillin and discharged 11 days later.
- A five-month-old girl in New Jersey was hospitalized because of vomiting, lethargy, and fever. She was treated and returned home after 10 days.
- Each of these children tested positive for salmonella bacteria, and all had been exposed to a reptile.

Most experts do not recommend having a pet reptile in homes where family members are younger than five. Whatever you decide, all experts recommend these reptile rules for those who own reptiles as pets:

- Always wash your hands with warm, soapy water after handling your animals or touching their cages.
- Never clean cages in the kitchen or anywhere you prepare food.
- Do not permit unsupervised handling of reptiles by children under 12.
- If you have open cuts or sores, cover them with bandages or wear rubber gloves before handling reptiles.
- Reptiles are not a good choice for day care centers.

A further thought: In the early 1970s, after thousands of infants and small children were diagnosed with turtle-related salmonella infection, the Federal Drug Administration banned the sale of baby turtles with shells four inches in length or less. The agency believed that turtles larger than four inches did not pose the same threat since children were not likely to try and fit them into their mouths.

Though the public is generally unaware of the ban, it is still in effect.

CHLAMYDIA INFECTION DURING PREGNANCY

Q *Early in this pregnancy, my doctor diagnosed a chlamydia infection and treated me with antibiotics. Can I assume the baby will be all right? If left untreated, how might chlamydia affect the baby?*

A If your infection was treated successfully, your baby should be fine. However, you should inform your baby's doctor about your medical history, just in case.

Untreated, mothers can pass a chlamydia infection to their babies as they pass through the birth canal at the time of delivery. It may cause an eye infection, but that is easily treated. More serious complications include pneumonia, which may require hospitalizing the baby.

IS THERE A CURE FOR GENITAL HERPES?

Q *I am one confused 17-year- old. My doctor says I have genital herpes, and it can't be cured. If that's true, why did he give me these pills? Also, since I'm pregnant, will the herpes harm my baby?*

A Your doctor is correct: There is no cure for genital herpes. The pills he prescribed help heal the sores sooner and may limit relapses.

Genital herpes is a highly contagious sexually transmitted disease. The cause is a strain of the herpes simplex virus. This virus enters your body through small breaks in your skin or mucus membranes. The illness consists of pain, itching, and sores in your genital area. Sexual intercourse is usually the primary way it spreads.

In adults, genital herpes generally doesn't cause any other permanent complications besides the sores. However, a woman with open sores can pass the infection on to her baby as the infant slides through the birth canal. When this happens, the baby may become seriously ill and suffer brain damage, blindness, or death.

To prevent the baby from coming into contact with the virus, a cesarean section is usually recommended. Unfortunately, even this approach doesn't always work.

A further thought: Each year in the United States, about 9,000 people are hospitalized for chickenpox and about 90 people die from the disease. The most common complication is a bacterial infection of the skin. The next most common problems are pneumonia and encephalitis, an infection of the brain.

When an adult gets chickenpox, the disease is usually more severe, often developing into pneumonia. Adults are almost 10 times more likely to be hospitalized for chickenpox than children under 14 years of age. Adults are also more than 20 times more likely to die from the disease. If a pregnant woman gets chickenpox, her unborn baby may have complications.

The American Academy of Pediatrics recommends a single dose of the chickenpox vaccine for all children between 12 and 18 months of age who have not had chickenpox.

Older children who have not had chickenpox and have not been immunized should be immunized with a single dose.

For healthy children older than 13, two doses of the vaccine are required, four to eight weeks apart.

DO CHILDHOOD EAR INFECTIONS NEED ANTIBIOTICS?

As most of you would probably guess, middle ear infections, technically known as acute otitis media, are the most commonly treated bacterial infections in children. But did you know that treatment for these infections accounts for more than 50 percent of all pediatric antibiotic prescriptions?

Now, let's make this a little harder. What would you guess is the total annual cost in this country for the millions of doses of antibiotics used to treat these bothersome ear infections?

- Is it $500 million?
- One billion?
- Two billion?
- Perhaps more?

The answer, my friends, is $5 billion annually, which amounts to $13.7 million daily. That's right, $13.7 million is spent every day in this country on antibiotics to treat middle ear infections in children.

Now, what would you say if I told you that several highly respected studies have shown that most cases of middle ear infection in children can be managed without antibiotics?

- You might say I don't know what I'm talking about.
- Or you might conclude that it's better to be safe than sorry and demand that your doctor treat your child's middle ear infection with antibiotics anyway.
- Or, if you have just spent $30 or more for a seven-day supply of antibiotics to treat your five-year-old's ear infection, you might wonder whether your hard-earned money couldn't be put to better use.

We all know by now about the increasing concern over the growing resistance of common bacteria to antibiotics. These concerns, combined with the potential side effects from antibiotics, led most physicians in Europe to adopt a different approach to treating ear infections than the one used by physicians in the United States. In Europe, physicians prescribe medications to make the child comfortable and reserve antibiotics for those children who don't recover right away.

More recently, a pediatrician in England has reported he was able to further decrease the use of antibiotics in his practice by giving parents of children with ear infections a "safety-net" antibiotic prescription for them to fill if symptoms did not resolve with observation and medicine for pain within 48 hours.

This latest approach to treating ear infections in children led researchers at the University of Cincinnati to do a study to find out if the safety-net approach to treating ear infections really works and if parents would accept it.

Of 194 children enrolled in the Cincinnati study, only 31 percent used their safety-net prescription.

Moreover, 63 percent of parents reported they would be willing to treat future middle ear infections with pain medication alone. The complete results of this study were published in *Pediatrics*, the official medical journal of the American Academy of Pediatrics.

The authors of the Cincinnati study were quick to point out two limitations to their study:

- The sample size was relatively small.
- Minority enrollment was lacking.

Before recommending their approach to others, they started a much larger study to see whether they can confirm the findings of their smaller study.

So what do you think?

- If your child came down with a middle ear infection, would you be willing to treat your child with pain medicine, while holding off on antibiotics for at least 48 hours, to see if the infection would resolve by itself?
- Or would you rather start antibiotics right away, realizing that in most cases the antibiotics aren't needed?

Of course, what you and I think may not matter if the safety-net approach to prescribing antibiotics catches on and becomes a standard of care. Then the insurance companies will have the final say.

LEARNING FROM THE SCARS OF CHICKENPOX

Talking to myself about chickenpox:

I: Remember when you had the chickenpox?
Me: Sure do. I can still see this pathetic little boy lying on the couch, covered with itchy bumps. Mom is sitting beside me, dabbing away with cotton balls soaked in calamine lotion.
I: Do you remember what she said?
Me: She said don't pick at the scabs. If you do, you'll be scarred for life.
I: Did you listen?
Me: No, they itched too much. I have the scars on my legs to prove it.
I: Any other complications?

Me: No. I was one of the lucky ones.
I: How so?
Me: Chickenpox is dangerous, not only for children, but also for adults. Only 10 percent of cases occur in adults, but they account for more than half the deaths.
I: What about the chickenpox vaccine? Doesn't it help?
Me: It's very effective. The trouble is lots of kids don't get it.
I: Why not?
Me: Some parents still think chickenpox is no big deal. Others worry about the vaccine's safety.
I: Is it safe?
Me: All vaccines carry some risk. But the risk of serious complications from chickenpox is much greater than the risk of complications from the vaccine.
I: So what do you tell parents?
Me: I tell them the chickenpox vaccine is recommended for children 12 to 18 months of age who have not had the chickenpox. Older, unvaccinated children, can be vaccinated at any visit. If you want to think about it and get more information, go to the American Academy of Pediatrics Web site (www.aap.org).
I: That's quite a speech.
Me: Sorry, I got carried away.
I: Anything else?
Me: Unvaccinated children, who have been exposed to a child with chickenpox, can still get protection if they get immunized within five days after first exposure. Within 72 hours is best.
I: And don't pick at the scabs?
Me: Right. Don't pick the scabs.

DEET IS BEST FOR FIGHTING MOSQUITOES

Q *My husband is taking our two children, ages five and seven, on a camping trip. With all the talk lately about West Nile Virus infections and Lyme disease, I'm worried about mosquito bites and ticks. Can you tell me if there's a safe lotion or spray that will protect them against these insects?*

A Browsing the aisles of your grocery or drug store, you can find a confusing array of lotions, creams, and sprays designed to keep pesky mosquitoes and ticks away from your husband and children. What does and doesn't work? Which one lasts the longest? What is safe for children?

Once you know your products, your choice is fairly simple. You should be looking for the safest, most effective, and longest-acting insect repellant for the money.

Last year, a study published in the *New England Journal of Medicine* showed that products containing DEET (N,N-diethyl-3-methylbenzamide) were the most effective in repelling mosquitoes for long periods of time.

More recently, the American Academy of Pediatrics issued a new policy stating that DEET-containing products are not only the most effective mosquito repellants available, but they are also effective against ticks. DEET, however, is not recommended for use in children under two months of age.

The concentration of DEET in insect repellants ranges from less than 10 percent to more than 30 percent. As the concentration increases, the duration of activity increases also.

For example, products with concentrations around 10 percent are effective for about two hours while products with concentrations of about 24 percent provide an average of five hours of protection. The safety of DEET does not appear to be related to differences in these concentrations.

A prudent approach is to select the product with the lowest concentration of DEET effective for the amount of time spent outdoors. Most experts recommend that you spray a DEET-containing aerosol on your clothing prior to going outdoors, and apply a DEET-containing cream on exposed skin. It's generally agreed that DEET should not be applied more than once a day.

Other precautions include the following:

- Apply DEET sparingly on exposed skin; do not use under clothing.
- Do not use DEET on the hands of young children: avoid applying to areas around the eyes and mouth.
- Do not use DEET over cuts, wounds, or irritated skin. Wash treated skin with soap and water after returning indoors; also wash treated clothing.
- Avoid spraying in enclosed areas; do not use DEET near food.

A further thought: In addition to mosquito and tick repellant, it makes sense to take other precautions against insect bites:

- Cover as much skin as possible with loose, light-colored clothing and a hat.
- Remove any standing water (the ideal breeding place for mosquitoes) from yards, campsites, and other outdoor areas as soon as possible.
- If you will be exposed to mosquitoes for long periods of time, consider using mosquito netting inside your tent.
- Some nets even come pretreated with repellant.

DO COUGH SUPPRESSANTS WORK IN CHILDREN WITH A COLD?

Here's the situation: Your three-year-old has had a cold for several days. Her breathing passages have reacted to the viral invasion by swelling and secreting mucus, accounting for her noisy breathing and her tell-tale runny nose. Mucus also pours inside, causing a postnasal drip, a throat tickle and an intermittent, hacking cough. During the day, her cough is tolerable, but as night falls, it gets much worse. Last night, she coughed so much that neither one of you got much sleep.

Bleary-eyed and confused, you survey the "cough and cold" shelf at your local pharmacy. Each of the decongestants and cough suppressants claim victory over secretions and cough. Which one should you choose?

Cough is probably the most bothersome symptom for children with upper respiratory infections. Each winter, a hacking cough that won't go away brings more children to the doctor than any other symptom.

The most popular over-the-counter cough and cold remedies contain dextromethorphan, abbreviated DM, or diphenhydramine, abbreviated DPH. During the winter months, medicines containing DM and DPH fly off pharmacy shelves.

The only problem is none of these medications have been shown conclusively to work in children, according to the American Academy of Pediatrics. So if you seem confused, think about the thousands of pediatricians who belong to the AAP and look to it for guidance.

In an attempt to clarify this confusion, researchers at the Pennsylvania State College of Medicine in Hershey, Pennsylvania, designed a study to answer two questions:

- Are commonly used over-the-counter medications that contain DM and DPH superior to placebo (a fake medicine) for the treatment of nocturnal cough and sleep difficulty associated with upper respiratory infections?
- Do parents have improved sleep quality when their children receive these medications when compared to a placebo?

It took the researchers a full year to enroll 100 children—ranging in age from 2 to 18, with a cough due to a cold—in their study. They excluded patients with asthma, pneumonia, croup, sinusitis, or allergic rhinitis (sneezing, itchy and watery eyes).

Each child was randomly assigned to receive one of three medications 30 minutes before bedtime as follows:

- 33 patients received a medication containing DM
- 33 patients received a medication containing DPH
- 34 patients received a simple syrup, the placebo

The medications were distributed by the pharmacy in a brown paper bag so that no one, except the pharmacist, knew which medication each child would be taking.

So, what do you think the researchers found?

All three treatment groups, including the placebo group, dramatically improved.

The kids coughed less, their coughs were less severe, they slept better, and so did their parents. In other words, those kids who took a simple syrup, the placebo, improved just as much as those who took DM or DPH.

Insomnia was reported more frequently in those children who were given DM while drowsiness was reported more frequently in those who received DPH.

So, back to our original question: Which medication do you choose? It's best to ask your doctor, or, at least, ask the pharmacist. The good news is that all products seem to work equally well, but mainly because we humans are programmed to see good results.

A further thought: Once upon a time, back when I was in medical school, Dr. John Krantz, our pharmacology professor, devoted an entire lecture to the art of prescription writing. He believed, in most cases, that the deliberate act of writing the prescription combined with a few words of encouragement did as much to relieve most patient's symptoms as the bottle of medicine itself. Call it the placebo effect or call it faith in your doctor. It works!

Skin conditions

WHAT TO DO ABOUT DIAPER RASH

Q *I can't seem to clear up my daughter's reddened and sore bottom for more than two or three weeks before it starts up again. Cornstarch helps, but when I stop using it, the redness reappears. Can you tell me what to do about this frustrating problem?*

A Most likely, your daughter has irritant contact dermatitis, the most common form of diaper rash. (Diaper rash is simply a general term for any rash or irritation in the area covered by the diaper.) Let me explain how rashes happen then we'll talk about treatment.

Normally, our skin forms a protective barrier against the outside world. When a wet diaper is left on too long, this protective barrier begins to swell and becomes more susceptible to injury.

When stool and urine interact, chemicals in the stool attack the skin, causing further swelling and injury. At this point, a baby's bottom may appear red and sore, like you described. Once the skin is damaged, continued exposure to urine and stool creates a vicious cycle that's difficult to break.

What to do about diaper rash? Consider the following guidelines:

- **Change your baby's diapers often.** Because prolonged contact with urine and stool causes diaper rash, change your baby's diaper as soon as possible

after she wets or soils. When practical, expose your baby's bottom to air.
- **Never use plastic pants; they hold moisture in.** Super-absorbent disposable diapers absorb up to 80 times their weight in liquid and keep urine away from the skin. Whatever type of diaper you use be sure the diaper doesn't fit too tightly.
- **Do not clean or wash excessively; this also irritates the skin.** When changing a wet diaper, only use warm water to rinse your baby's skin. After a bowel movement, clean the diaper area gently using warm water and a small amount of mild soap such as Dove, Johnson's Ultra Sensitive, or a Cetaphil cleansing bar. Be sure to rinse away all of the soap. It's best not to use diaper wipes when your baby has a rash.
- **Consider using a barrier ointment to keep urine and stool away from the skin.** Choices include A&D ointment, Balmex, Desitin, Johnson & Johnson diaper ointment, or Triple Paste. Cornstarch can also be used.

If your baby's diaper rash doesn't respond within three days or seems to be getting worse, make an appointment to see your doctor.

A further thought: Victor Mills, a Proctor & Gamble researcher, came up with the idea for a disposable diaper in 1956 while baby-sitting for his granddaughter. It seems he strongly disliked changing and washing cloth diapers and decided to do something about it.

Three years later, Proctor & Gamble test-marketed 37,000 handmade Pampers, which were fastened with safety pins, in Rochester, New York.

Today, disposable diaper sales in the United States exceed $4 billion each year.

Victor Mills died in 1996 at the ripe old age of 100.

RECOGNIZING AND TREATING CRADLE CAP

Q *The back of my baby's scalp has a patch of yellowish, crusty material that flakes off and is hard to remove. Can you tell me what it is and how to get rid of it?*

A Most likely, your baby has cradle cap, also called seborrhea, which is very common in infants. It's caused by too much oil, which crusts over and may irritate the skin. It usually begins in the first weeks of life and slowly disappears over a period of weeks or months.

The best treatment is daily washing with soap and water. You can soften the crust by rubbing with baby oil or petroleum jelly. Then wash the scalp with a mild shampoo and pat dry. Brush it out with a soft brush or toothbrush. If you follow this routine, it should do the trick.

Stronger medicated shampoos may loosen the crust more quickly, but use them only after consulting your doctor. If the crusting persists, your doctor may prescribe a cortisone cream or lotion. One percent hydrocortisone cream is a commonly used preparation.

WHAT ARE MONGOLIAN SPOTS?

Q *Our grandson was born with dark spots over his lower back. The doctor called them mongolian spots, but he never said what they were or what to expect later on. Can you tell me whether they are something to worry about? Will they eventually disappear?*

A Mongolian spots are areas of increased pigmentation often found on the lower back and buttocks of African-American, Asian, and Indian babies. They also occur in 5 to 10 percent of Caucasian babies. They fade during childhood but may not completely disappear. Otherwise, they have no clinical significance.

A further thought: Unfortunately, mongolian spots have been mistaken for bruises, raising a suspicion of child abuse. You might want to make a copy of your question and my response and give it to your grandson's parents, just in case.

ARE THESE THE BRUISES OF CHILD ABUSE?

Q *Recently, a police officer and a social worker from Children's Services showed up at our front door. They were responding to an anonymous complaint from the day care center where we take our 13-month-old daughter. Someone there had called Children's Services about "bruises" on my daughter's back. The officer wanted to know if we had been abusing our child.*

Before it was all over, we had to hire a lawyer and get our pediatrician involved. He went to court and testified that the so-called bruises were really mongolian spots that had been there from birth.

I hope this letter will help overzealous day care workers think twice before they put innocent families through the living hell we've been through.

A Unfortunately, in today's society, some people assume child abuse lurks around every corner, instead of using common sense. Had the concerned day care worker asked you about the "bruises," you could have explained your daughter's skin condition and asked your doctor for written verification. End of story.

Or, had you imagined your daughter's skin condition might be mistaken for bruises and raise a suspicion of child abuse, you could have explained her condition and

Walking the Baby Beat

obtained written verification when you first signed her up for day care. Another end to the story.

To avoid a misdiagnosis that can profoundly affect a child and her family, let's discuss two conditions, one you have already mentioned, that have been mistaken for the bruises of child abuse:

- *Mongolian spots* are irregular areas of increased pigmentation usually, but not always, found over the lower back and buttocks at birth. They're common in African-American, Hispanic, and Asian babies, but they also occur in Caucasian babies. Mongolian spots usually fade over time, but may not completely disappear. Otherwise, they're harmless.
- *Photodermatitis* is a visible skin reaction to light after a child has come into contact with certain plants. The skin reaction, which may resemble finger or handprints, occurs several hours to days after exposure to the plant. If the skin blisters, it may resemble a burn that has resulted from scalding. The correct diagnosis is suggested by taking a careful history and carefully examining the skin.

A further thought: Clothing dyes, such as the dye from a new pair of blue jeans, may rub off on a child's legs and be mistaken for the bruises of child abuse. In one such case, a child's parents were falsely accused of child abuse after their 18-month-old developed "bruises" on his legs. However, when the discolored area was rubbed with an alcohol swab, the so-called bruises disappeared and so did the accusation.

MOST HEMANGIOMAS DON'T NEED TREATMENT

Q *Our six-month-old son was born with a birthmark the size of a dime on his back; now, it's the size of a quarter. Our* *pediatrician called it a strawberry hemangioma and said it would get bigger before it got smaller and disappeared. But it's hard just watching it grow. What can you tell us about this problem? Is there anything more we should do?*

A As your doctor predicted, the small clump of blood vessels, known as a strawberry hemangioma, has gotten larger. Most likely, it will continue to grow until he's two or three. Then it will start to turn gray, from the in-growth of normal skin cells, and eventually disappear.

A strawberry hemangioma should only be treated if it interferes with a vital function, such as seeing or eating, or if it becomes irritated or infected. Because your son's hemangioma is located out of harm's way, on his back, taking a wait-and-see attitude seems appropriate. Reassurance and regular checkups should do the trick.

WHAT'S THE DIFFERENCE BETWEEN IMPETIGO AND RINGWORM?

Q *I hate to sound so dumb, but can you explain the difference between impetigo and ringworm?*

A Impetigo is a bacterial infection of the skin. It often starts as a pimple on the face that breaks open from rubbing. A scab or crust, partly brown, partly honey-colored, soon follows. Scabs or crusts may then show up on other parts of the body, carried there by the child's hands.

Impetigo is usually not a serious medical problem, but it spreads easily if neglected, and it is contagious. A child with impetigo should see a doctor for diagnosis and treatment. If caught early, a local antibiotic ointment may do the trick. Otherwise, the child may need a course of antibiotics.

Ringworm, on the other hand, is a fungal infection of the skin. It starts out small and gradually enlarges to nickel-sized, circular patches of reddened, scaly skin with a smooth, clear center. Ringworm of the scalp consists of round patches of scaly skin in which the hair is broken off. Ringworm is mildly contagious and requires diagnosis and treatment by a doctor.

You can help prevent ringworm by identifying and treating any pets with the problem. Look for scaling, itchy, hairless areas on your dog or cat, and have them treated right away.

WHAT CAUSES THE RASH OF POISON IVY?

Q *Our five-year-old daughter has poison ivy. Can you explain what causes the rash and the best way to treat it? Is poison ivy contagious?*

A The rash of poison ivy—as well as that of poison oak and poison sumac—is caused by an allergic reaction to the oil in the poison ivy plant. The rash occurs from several hours to three days after contact with the plant and begins in the form of blisters, which are accompanied by severe itching.

Contrary to popular belief, the rash is not spread by the fluid in the blisters. It is spread when small amounts of oil remain under the child's fingernails, on her clothing, or on a pet's hair; and that oil comes into contact with other parts of her body.

The rash will not spread to another person unless the oil that remains also comes into contact with that person's skin. In other words, if the oil from the plant remains on a child's body or clothes, the child may act like a walking poison ivy plant.

The American Academy of Pediatrics recommends the following approach to treating poison ivy:

- After a child has come into contact with poison ivy, poison oak, or poison sumac, wash all clothes in soap and water. Also, wash the area of skin that was

exposed, as well as the child's hands, with soap and water for at least 10 minutes.
- If the rash is mild, apply calamine lotion three or four times a day to cut down on the itching.
- Topical 1 percent hydrocortisone cream can be applied to decrease inflammation.
- If the rash is severe, on the face, or on extensive parts of the body, see your doctor.

Your doctor should also be called if you notice any of the following:

- A severe eruption that doesn't respond to the previously described home methods.
- Any evidence of infection, such as blistering, redness, or oozing.
- Your child develops a fever.

Abdominal disorders

WHAT IS AN INTUSSUSCEPTION?

Q *My sister's three-month-old had stomach pain and then some blood in her stool. At the hospital, the doctor did a barium enema for what he called an intussusception. After that, she was fine. Can you explain how this condition occurs? How did the barium enema help relieve her problem?*

A Intussusception is an uncommon, but life-threatening condition, in which the intestine "telescopes" into itself and becomes obstructed.

Typically, a healthy, well-fed baby between 3 and 36 months of age has the sudden onset of colicky abdominal pain. The infant draws her legs up in pain then completely relaxes between episodes. Over several hours, the child begins vomiting and her abdomen becomes distended. In half the cases, bloody stools are passed. Occasionally, intussusception occurs in the newborn period.

An emergency barium enema serves two purposes:

- It makes the diagnosis, which the radiologist can see on the monitoring screen.
- It frequently reduces the obstruction. When it doesn't reduce the obstruction, the child is taken immediately to surgery.

Because intussusception in older children is often associated with lymphosarcoma, a deadly form of cancer, exploratory surgery is usually recommended when an intussusception occurs in a child over six years of age.

A further thought: Though newborns see all colors of the spectrum at birth, they can't distinguish the blue color spectrum (greens, violets, blues) or pastels very well. By about four months of age, babies are able to see a full range of color. A baby's overall sight is fully matured by one year of age.

WHAT IS NECROTIZING ENTEROCOLITIS?

Q *My sister's little girl was born six weeks premature and weighed almost four pounds. She had breathing problems but soon got over that. But when the doctors tried to feed her, she came down with an intestinal problem. I believe my sister called it NEC.*

The doctors had to operate and take out part of her intestine to save her life. After she recovered from the surgery, the doctors tried again to feed her. This time she did fine. She's going home soon and seems to be doing great.

D. Gary Benfield, M.D.

Can you explain what happened to my little niece to cause her to have surgery? Can it come back again?

A Necrotizing enterocolitis, also known as NEC, is a disease that most often affects premature infants; however, some term or close-to-term infants can also get it. NEC occurs when the following sequence of events takes place:

- Blood supplying the baby's intestine is decreased or interrupted.
- This decreased blood supply, in turn, decreases or interrupts the amount of oxygen delivered to the intestine.
- Lack of oxygen causes damage to an area of the intestinal wall.

Similarly, when the blood supply to an area of the heart is decreased or interrupted, the heart muscle is deprived of adequate oxygen, resulting in muscle damage and a heart attack. Or, when the blood supply to an area of the brain is compromised, and the patient's brain is damaged from a lack of oxygen, it is called a stroke. Thus, the underlying mechanism that produces tissue damage when the blood supply to any organ is decreased or interrupted is the same.

Now, back to our story.

- When an area of the intestinal wall is damaged from a lack of oxygen, bacteria that are normally present within the intestine invade the intestinal wall, causing further damage.
- Intestinal damage may be minimal or quite extensive, depending on several factors.
- In severe cases, the wall of the intestine may perforate or rupture, leading to an infection of the abdominal cavity known as peritonitis.

Similar to a case of appendicitis in an older child, the surgeon faced with a critically ill, premature baby with NEC would like to operate and remove the damaged area of the intestine before it perforates and peritonitis sets in.

It sounds like the doctors operated in time and only had to remove a small section of your niece's intestine. It also sounds like your niece has had a nice recovery.

After the baby goes home, your sister will need to watch her closely. Any patient, young or old, who has had abdominal surgery has a small risk of developing adhesions at the operative site. I'm sure the baby's doctors will explain what to look for, just in case. Otherwise, the risk of another bout of NEC is extremely low.

A further thought: Occasionally, when NEC is severe and involves an extensive section of intestine, the amount of healthy intestine remaining after surgery may be quite short and unable to absorb enough nutrients and water from feedings. This condition is called the short bowel syndrome or "short gut." Babies with a short gut may require intravenous nutrition for months or even years. Unfortunately, some of these children don't survive.

ABDOMINAL PAIN AND VOMITING: A NEW TWIST

A six-year-old girl is your next patient. She is with her mother who made the appointment this morning.

They give a four-day history of intermittent vomiting and abdominal pain. Four days ago, she was seen in the emergency room where she was diagnosed as having a "virus" and given a rectal suppository.

The next day, her parents took her back to the ER because of continued vomiting and pain. A urinalysis was "suspicious," and she was started on an antibiotic for a suspected urinary tract infection.

A day later, her mother took her to an urgent care center. The doctor suspected constipation and prescribed treatment with enemas. The enemas produced a good amount of stool, but there was no change in the girl's abdominal pain and vomiting.

She describes the pain as crampy and says it comes and goes. When she vomits, it's clear-colored, not green or streaked with blood.

The girl's temperature is slightly elevated, but her vital signs are normal. When you listen to her chest, her lungs are clear and her heart sounds are normal. Her abdomen is soft to the touch, and she has normally active bowel sounds. But she is tender over her lower abdomen.

The child seems to have something more significant going on than a virus or constipation. You order some tests and think about the possibilities:

- Her white blood cell count is elevated, but her urinalysis is normal. A call to the emergency room reveals that the urine culture obtained three days ago was negative. It's unlikely that she has a urinary tract infection.
- Appendicitis typically starts with the acute onset of vomiting and abdominal pain. Her fever and the elevated white count are consistent with this diagnosis. Did she have appendicitis that perforated and formed an abscess?
- Bowel obstruction could start in this way, but she has produced stools within the past 24 hours. She's not distended and she doesn't look sick enough for complete bowel obstruction.

You admit her to the hospital and make arrangements for an ultrasound of her abdomen and pelvis.

The ultrasound makes the diagnosis. A pelvic mass is seen pushing on the right side of her urinary bladder. Torsion or twisting of the right ovary seems most likely.

Walking the Baby Beat

Your patient is taken to surgery, where the surgeon discovers a large, swollen, hemorrhagic ovary and twisted fallopian tube, which he removes. Her post-op course goes smoothly, and she is discharged from the hospital in good condition.

Torsion or twisting of the ovary is uncommon in young girls, but it can occur at any age, even in newborns. Most cases are associated with ovarian cysts or other tumors. But they also occur in normal ovaries, which was true in this case.

The child typically presents to a doctor with abdominal pain, with or without vomiting. Because the right ovary is most commonly involved, preoperatively the diagnosis of acute appendicitis is often made. But at surgery, the surgeon is often surprised.

Why does the normal ovary twist in this way? No one knows. But torsion or twisting of the ovary should always be kept in mind when one is considering the possibility of appendicitis or any acute abdominal event in a female.

Early diagnosis and surgery may save the ovary. Unfortunately, in almost all reported cases, surgery came too late, and the ovary had to be removed.

Child safety

A SWALLOWED COIN CAN BE DANGEROUS

Q *Our 17-month-old recently picked up a penny from the coffee table, put it in his mouth, and gulped it down. It happened so fast there was nothing I could do. I took him to emergency, and the doctor took an X-ray. It was there in his stomach. The doctor said to check his bowel movements and sent us home. Do you know how long it takes for a coin to pass out the other end?*

A When a child swallows a coin, it usually takes about five days before you see the change. By the way, it was important for the doctor to locate the coin by taking an X-ray. Once a swallowed coin makes it to the stomach, it usually passes through the digestive tract without difficulty. But if it gets stuck in the esophagus or the child chokes and the coin winds up in the windpipe, things can get complicated. Then the coin must be removed under emergency conditions using special techniques.

ARE INFANT WALKERS TOO DANGEROUS?

Q *I'd like to buy a walker for our nine-month-old son to help him learn to walk, but my wife disagrees. She says walkers are too dangerous. I think she's worried over nothing. Can you help settle our disagreement?*

A Here are two myths about infant walkers:

- They help babies learn to walk sooner.
- They are safe.

According to medical research, walkers may actually slow the process of learning to walk. Walkers do strengthen the muscles in the lower legs, but they don't strengthen those in the upper legs and hips, muscles used most in walking.

Walkers may also eliminate the desire to walk, because they allow children to get around easily.

They may also hinder the walking development of babies who have motor delays by teaching them abnormal movement patterns.

The government estimates that more than 28,000 injuries related to walker accidents are treated annually in hospital emergency rooms. Babies in walkers can sustain serious head injuries if they tumble down stairways or steps between levels. They can turn over in walkers snagged by cords, door thresholds, and carpet edges; roll themselves against hot stoves and heaters; fall over concrete curbs; or tumble into swimming pools.

As it turns out, walkers are one of the most dangerous of baby products, according to Consumer's Union. Both the American Academy of Pediatrics and Consumers Union strongly urge parents not to use them.

I'll side with your wife on this one.

A further thought: Here are some gentle reminders to help keep your baby safe:

- Never leave your baby unattended in water. If you need to answer the phone or otherwise interrupt a bath, wrap your baby in a towel and take her with you.
- Never heat a baby's formula or food in the microwave oven. Hot spots might burn him.
- Never hang a pacifier by a string around your baby's neck. You create the risk of strangling.

DO SWIMMING LESSONS PREVENT DROWNING?

Q *I've enrolled my two-year-old in a summer swimming class so he can have fun and learn to swim, and I can relax when he's around the water. But when I mentioned my plan to his pediatrician, she said he's too young and went on and on about the danger involved. Did I do the wrong thing or is my doctor overreacting?*

A You did nothing wrong. However, you should never relax—swimming lessons or not—when your child is around water. Why? Because studies show that swimming lessons don't protect young children from drowning.

Most experts believe that children aren't developmentally ready for formal swimming lessons until after their fourth birthday. This recommendation doesn't mean that summer swimming programs for infants and toddlers have no value; they certainly do. But it does mean that these programs should not be promoted as a way to decrease the risk of drowning. Parents should not feel secure that their child is safe in the water or safe from drowning just because the child has participated in such a program.

Experienced life guards tell us that young children who are drowning rarely thrash around or fight for their lives. They simply go under and don't come up. You don't hear any yelling or screaming; it's pretty quick.

It's important for parents to stay within arm's reach of young children when in or around water, even if the youngsters have taken swimming classes. No swimming program is an adequate substitute for constant adult supervision. And supervision doesn't mean an adult can sit in a lawn chair and watch the kids from poolside. You must be within arm's reach at all times, providing "touch supervision."

A further thought: In the United States, drowning rates are highest among children ages one through two years. In Arizona, California, Florida, and Texas, drowning is the leading cause of death in this age group.

DOES THIS CRIB MEET MODERN SAFETY STANDARDS?

Q *My wife and I will soon be new grandparents and are very excited. We have a 25-year-old crib and wonder whether it is possible to make it safe to use when our grandchild visits. If it's not safe, how should I dispose of it so no one else will use it and endanger their own baby.*

Walking the Baby Beat

A A crib manufactured before 1985 may not meet current safety standards. Because you have an older crib, inspect it carefully for the following features:

- Slats should be no more than 2 ⅜ inches apart so a child's head cannot become trapped between them.
- There should be no cutouts in the headboard or footboard, as your grandchild's head could become trapped in them.
- If the crib has corner posts (sometimes called finials), unscrew them or cut them off. Loose clothing can become snagged on these and choke a baby.
- Make sure all screws, bolts, and hardware are tightly in place to prevent the crib from coming apart. Check these features regularly; an active child can cause screws, bolts, and other hardware to loosen.
- Many older cribs were painted with lead-based paint, which can poison children if they gnaw on the crib rails (it does happen). As a precaution, you can strip the old paint and then repaint the crib using high-quality, new enamel. Then place plastic strips (available at most children's furniture stores) over the top of the side rails.

You can prevent other crib hazards by observing the following guidelines:

- If you purchase a new mattress, remove and destroy all plastic wrapping material that comes with it. If you cover the mattress with heavy plastic, be sure the cover fits tightly; zippered covers are best.
- The mattress should fit snugly so your grandchild cannot slip into the crack between it and the crib side. If you can insert more than two fingers

between the mattress and the sides or ends of the crib, replace the mattress with one that fits snugly.
- Use a crib bumper when your grandchild is an infant. Be sure the pad goes all the way around the crib and is secured with at least six straps or ties, to keep the bumper from falling away from the sides. To prevent strangulation, the ties should be no more than six inches long.
- As soon as your grandchild can pull to a standing position, remove crib bumpers as well as any toys, pillows, or stuffed animals that are large enough to be used as a step for climbing out.
- If you hang a mobile over your grandchild's crib, be sure it is securely attached to the side rails. Hang it high enough so the baby cannot reach it to pull it down. Remove it when he is able to get up on his hands and knees, or when he reaches five months, whichever comes first.

What should you do with your 25-year-old crib if it's not safe, and you don't want someone else to take a chance and use it? Take it apart and remove all of the hardware. Then either break it up for firewood or ask your trash collector to haul the parts away.

GRIM REALITY OF MISSING AND ABDUCTED CHILDREN

Q *Can you explain the difference between a runaway child and a thrownaway child? Do you have any information about what happens to children when they are abducted by people from outside the family?*

A In order to answer your first question, we must first turn to Congress. In 1984, Congress passed the Missing Children's Assistance Act. This legislation requires the U.S. Department of Justice to conduct periodic national surveys to determine the incidence of children reported missing as well as those who were recovered for that particular year. In the most recent survey, conducted in 1999, surveyors defined a runaway and a thrownaway child in the following way:

- **Runaway:** A child leaves home without permission and stays away overnight; or a child 14 years or younger who is away from home chooses not to return and stays away overnight; or a child 15 years or older stays away two nights.
- **Thrownaway:** A child is asked or told to leave (or prevented from returning home) by a parent or other household adult, no adequate alternative care is arranged, and the child is out of the household overnight.

The 1999 survey found that more than 1.6 million children were runaways or thrownaways that year, for an average of 4,400 each day.

Now for your second question about nonfamily abductions: The 1999 survey also found that some 58,000 additional children, an average of 159 per day, were victims of nonfamily abductions.

Definition: A nonfamily abduction was defined as a nonfamily perpetrator takes a child, or detains a child for at least one hour in an isolated place, by the use of force or threat of bodily harm, and without parent permission.

Of the 58,000 victims of nonfamily abductions, 99 percent were returned home, but almost half had been sexually assaulted.

Most of these victims were adolescents, broken down by age as follows:

- 59 percent were between 15 and 17 years old
- 22 percent were between 12 and 14 years old
- 12 percent were between 6 and 11 years old
- 7 percent were less than 5 years of age

Perpetrators of nonfamily abductions break down as follows:

- 45 percent were described as a stranger
- 21 percent were described as an acquaintance
- 17 percent were described as a friend

Other perpetrators included baby-sitters, caretakers, neighbors, or persons of authority.

In 1999, 115 of these cases involved a stereotypical kidnapping, defined as a nonfamily abduction in which a child is detained overnight, transported at least 50 miles, held for ransom, abducted with intent to keep the child permanently, or killed.

- In 40 percent of those 115 episodes, the abducted child was killed, and 4 percent were not recovered.
- According to a report issued by the U.S. Attorney General, the typical murder victim of a nonfamily abduction is just over 11 years of age.
- In most cases the initial contact between victim and killer is within a quarter mile of the victim's home.
- Some 76 percent of victims are female. The youngest female victims (1–5 years old) tend to be killed by friends or acquaintances, while older female victims (over 16) tend to be killed by strangers.
- In contrast, male victims of all ages tend to be killed by strangers.

Most killers in child abduction cases are motivated by sexual assault. Typically, the murderer of an abducted child is an unmarried male, 27 years of age, who lives alone or with his parents. Almost two-thirds have a history of violent crime and that history often includes rape or other sexual assaults involving children.

PREVENTING ABDUCTION: A GUIDE FOR PARENTS

The following age-appropriate suggestions of some things parents can do to make their child a difficult target for kidnappers and sexual predators is furnished by the National Center for Missing and Exploited Children (www.missingkids.org) and the KlaasKids Foundation (www.klaaskids.org). These suggestions may be photocopied and distributed to parents and their children.

A preschooler should:

- always be under the direct supervision of an adult.
- be taught his (her) full name, address, and phone number and how to dial 911.
- if lost, seek assistance of a uniformed police officer, store cashier, or a woman with a child.
- always ask your permission before accepting a gift or going somewhere with someone else.

A school-age child should:

- always use the buddy system, taking a friend along when going somewhere.
- let you know where he is and where he is going, and his approximate times of arrival and departure.
- keep a safe distance (10 feet or more) from a car with someone in it, and never get into a car unless you have given permission to do so.
- be informed that adults do not need to ask a child for directions or for help finding a lost animal or child.
- never tell a phone caller that you aren't home or open the door if someone knocks if he is home alone. A latchkey child also needs to know who to call in an emergency.

- scream "No" or yell "Fire" when threatened. Such action immediately attracts attention and is an effective maneuver for thwarting an abductor.
- if followed, run to a safe place, a store, or anywhere there are lots of people.

A teenager should:

- continue to use the buddy system when going anywhere and let you know where she is. (Consider providing a cell phone to a responsible teenager, to make it easier for her to communicate her whereabouts to you.)
- be made aware that drugs and alcohol impair judgment and reaction time, rendering a person more susceptible to exploitation.
- check out the house before entering when arriving home; lock the door behind her; and call you to let you know when she arrives.
- never tell a phone caller that you are not home.

A further thought: Have you ever wondered whether those photo cards you get in the mail really help recover missing children? If you have, the answer is absolutely. One in six of the missing kids featured on those cards are recovered as a direct result of the photographs that reach up to 79 million homes weekly, according to the National Center for Missing and Exploited Children.

CRAWLING INFANTS LEAD DANGEROUS LIVES

Q *Our seven-month-old acts like he'll start to crawl any day now. So far, we've done well keeping him safe. I put him to sleep on his back, use a rear-facing infant seat when riding in the car, and never leave him alone at bath time. But I worry a bit about the things we should do to childproof the*

Walking the Baby Beat

house before he learns to crawl. Can you give us some advice, so we'll be prepared when he does start to crawl?

A Let's get down on our hands and knees and crawl around your house, pretending we're your son, who's learning to crawl. Let's also pretend your son can talk to himself. He's crawling around on the living room carpet right now while you fix dinner:

"This is so much fun. I love how the carpet feels against my knees. What's this shiny thing? It looks like a paper clip. Wonder how it tastes. Ouch, it hurt my tooth. I'll leave it here and head over to the wall.

"What's this thing on the wall? Dad said not to touch it, I might get shocked. Maybe I'll go back and get the paper clip and touch it with that. Oh, what the heck, it's too far away.

"The fireplace looks interesting. Let's see what's over there.

"It feels nice and warm here. The fire looks like fun. What's this? Dad used this box of stick matches to start the fire. Wonder how they taste? Ugh. No thanks.

"Maybe I'll head for the kitchen and see what mom is doing.

"What's this? A peanut on the floor. Wonder how it tastes? Oops. Swallowed it. Hope mom didn't see me do it.

"Where's mom? She must have gone to the bathroom. Let's see what's inside this open cupboard door.

"My, my. This sure looks like fun. There's dishwasher soap, Brillo pads, trash bags, and a mouse trap. Wonder what would happen if I touch it? Let me see.

"Ouch, ouch, ouch, ouch! Mommy, wherever you are please help me. My finger's caught in the trap, and it hurts so bad!"

Well, I think you get the message: Infants learning to crawl lead dangerous lives. No matter how many safety gadgets you buy, no matter how much you childproof your home, *the most important safety device is surveillance.* Gadgets are no substitute for your eyes and ears.

Of course you should also do the following:

- Put outlet covers over unused outlets or block them with furniture.
- Stow logs, matches, and fireplace tools out of reach.
- Move cleaning agents, medicines, vitamins, toiletries, mothballs, and other potentially toxic items out of reach or lock them up.
- Remove mobiles and hanging toys from his crib.
- Install gates to block stairways at bottom and top.
- Use doorstops and door holders to protect his fingers.
- Always keep your purse or a visitor's purse out of reach.

A further thought: You'll have to reevaluate these precautionary measures as your son grows up. Childproofing is an ongoing process. The gate you put at the top of the stairs for your eight-month-old may become his favorite climbing wall when he's two.

IS IT SAFE TO BURN CANDLES IN YOUR BEDROOM?

Q *I'm 16 and enjoy the scent of burning candles when I study at night in my room. I think I'm old enough to light a candle or two and not burn the house down. But my mom gets all hyper and makes me put them out. My dad is pretty cool about it and sides with me. Mom said to ask you, and she will go along with what you think. So should I be allowed to burn candles in my room or not?*

A I consulted with Sparky the Fire Dog, spokesdog for the National Fire Protection Association or NFPA, to help me answer your question. Sparky asked me to pass along these tips to help you use candles safely at home:

- Never burn a candle in the bedroom.
- Make sure a grown-up is always in the room when a candle is burning.
- If a grown-up leaves the room, make sure he or she puts out the candle first.
- Keep candles away from things that can catch fire, such as clothing, books, paper, curtains, Christmas trees, or decorations.
- Place candles on stable furniture in sturdy holders that won't tip over and are big enough to collect dripping wax.
- Don't place candles in windows, where they may ignite blinds or curtains.
- If the power goes out, have flashlights on hand to use instead of candles.

My final answer?

Take Sparky's advice and don't burn candles in your bedroom. Perhaps you could light a candle at the kitchen table—when one of your parents is nearby—and study there occasionally.

A further thought: Candles have become very popular, especially around the holidays. According to the National Candle Association, 7 out of 10 households now use candles. Unfortunately, this popularity has led to an increase in candle-caused fires.

New data from NFPA show candles started fires in 18,000 homes in 2001, for an average of 49 candle fires a day, a 15 percent increase from 2000, and more than triple the number in 1990.

In 2001, candle fires in the home were responsible for 190 deaths, 1,450 injuries, and $265 million in property damage. Forty-one percent of those fires were caused by burning candles in the bedroom; 11 percent started after someone fell asleep.

D. Gary Benfield, M.D.

Day care

WHAT HEALTH PROBLEMS EXCLUDE A CHILD FROM DAY CARE?

Q *I am about to open a day care center. Has any reputable organization published a list of health problems that exclude children from attending day care?*

A The American Academy of Pediatrics recommends the following criteria for excluding children from day care. Parents might also find these criteria helpful.

- Illness that prevents the child from comfortably participating in program activities.
- Illness that results in a greater need for care than what the staff can provide without compromising the health and safety of other children.
- Fever, lethargy, irritability, persistent crying, difficulty breathing, or other manifestations of possible severe illness.
- Diarrhea or stools that contain blood or mucus.
- E. coli or Shigella infection, until diarrhea resolves and two stool cultures are negative for these organisms.
- Vomiting two or more times in 24 hours, unless the vomiting is caused by a noncommunicable condition and the child is not in danger of dehydration.
- Mouth sores associated with drooling, unless the child's physician or local health department authority states that the child is not infectious.
- Rash with fever or behavior change, until a physician has determined that the illness is not a communicable disease.
- Purulent conjunctivitis (defined as pink or red conjunctiva with white or yellow discharge, often with

matted eyelids after sleep and eye pain or redness of the eyelids or surrounding skin), until examined by a physician and approved for readmission, with treatment.
- Tuberculosis, until the child's physician or local health department authority states that the child is not infectious.
- Impetigo, until 24 hours after treatment has been started.
- Strep throat, until 24 hours after treatment has been started.
- Head lice, until after the first treatment.
- Scabies, until after treatment has been given.
- Chickenpox, until all pustules have dried and crusted (usually six days).
- Whooping cough, until five days of appropriate antibiotic treatment (which is to be given for a total of 14 days) has been completed.
- Mumps, until nine days after onset of parotid gland swelling.
- Measles, until four days after onset of rash.
- Hepatitis A virus infection, until one week after onset of illness or jaundice (if symptoms are mild).

Child abuse

IT'S NEVER OKAY TO SHAKE A BABY

Q *Our neighbor's baby was recently rushed to the hospital and treated for convulsions. Later, the police arrested our neighbor and charged him with child abuse. The doctors discovered the baby had suffered brain damage from bleeding in his brain. They said our neighbor shook his son to try and stop his crying. Can you tell me how shaking a baby damages* *a baby's brain? For someone who has come very close to shaking his baby too, how can I keep from making the same mistake?*

A You have just described the shaken baby syndrome, a variety of serious injuries that can occur when a child is shaken.

A baby has very weak neck muscles that can't support its relatively heavy head. When a baby is shaken, its fragile brain moves back and forth within the skull. This movement can damage the eyes, spinal cord, and brain, causing seizures, delay in development, and even death.

Shaken baby syndrome is a form of child abuse. It usually happens when a parent or other caregiver shakes a baby because the baby won't stop crying. The American Academy of Pediatrics cautions, "If you've tried to calm your crying child but nothing seems to work, it's important to control your temper." If you feel as though you could lose control, the AAP suggests the following:

- Take a deep breath and count to 10.
- Take time out and let your baby cry alone.
- Call someone close to you for emotional support.
- Call your pediatrician or family doctor. A medical issue may be the reason your child is crying.

Remember: It's never okay to shake a baby.

SHAKEN BABY CASES CAN BE DIFFICULT TO PROVE

Q *I get so frustrated when these young men who have obviously shaken a baby, causing the baby's death, are found innocent and set free. Can't something be done to stop these miscarriages of justice?*

Walking the Baby Beat

A A wise judge once told me that just because a jury finds a defendant not guilty doesn't necessarily mean the defendant is innocent. It simply means the prosecutor failed to convince the jury otherwise.

So, yes, sometimes the accused in a shaken baby case does go free even though the autopsy clearly shows a badly damaged brain; even though experts link the damaged brain to violent shaking; even though the prosecutor thinks she has a clear-cut case; and even though you think so too.

By now, all of us should know that shaking can kill a baby. And if shaking doesn't kill the baby, it can cause brain damage, learning problems, cerebral palsy, seizures, and blindness. How does this happen? Shaking slams a baby's brain against the skull, causing bleeding outside and inside the brain.

But, consider this point: Many of us, from time to time, have gotten angry with our children. And many of us have lost control and spanked them, shaken them, or worse. So when a jury hears a shaken baby case, deep in the back of their minds they may think, "There, but for the grace of God, go I." All it takes is for one member of the jury to sympathize with the defendant and hold out, based on reasonable doubt.

Here's a case to show how doubt can be created.

A single mother goes out in the middle of the night to buy a pack of cigarettes, leaving her boyfriend behind with her baby. When she returns, she finds the boyfriend asleep on the couch and her baby close to death in his crib. Desperate to save her baby, she shakes him, and then calls 9-1-1. Later, the baby dies in the hospital and her boyfriend is indicted for murder.

The baby had been born prematurely and stayed in the hospital for several weeks with breathing problems. More than once, the mother was told that hers was a fragile baby.

Her boyfriend's attorney suggests to the jury that this fragile baby may have been on the verge of dying from

SIDS when his mother intervened. Naturally, she shook her baby. What mother wouldn't? And this act, not anything her boyfriend might have done, caused the hemorrhage found at autopsy.

When called to testify about the baby's autopsy, the medical examiner explains in meticulous detail why the baby's brain was already damaged before his mother found him, and other experts agree. But one juror still has doubt, and the defendant is set free.

This case shows why prosecutors should leave no stone unturned when they investigate a shaken baby case. Suppose, for instance, the prosecutor had dug deeper and interviewed the nurses who had cared for the baby in the hospital where he was born.

Suppose those nurses had testified that the boyfriend had been rough with the baby in the hospital and had frequently gotten angry with the baby, cursing him in their presence. Their testimony might have been enough to change that single juror's mind.

WAS THIS CHILD'S INJURY REALLY ACCIDENTAL?

Q *A friend of mine's two-year-old daughter recently fell down the stairs at home and was rushed to the hospital. Suspecting internal injuries, the doctors operated and found a hole in the small intestine, just beyond the stomach. The child recovered and is doing fine. But while the child was in the hospital, her mother was questioned several times by Child Protective Services because the doctors suspected child abuse. Fortunately, they didn't take the child away. Doesn't it seem logical that a fall down the stairs could cause such an injury?*

A To help answer your question, let me tell you about a study that was published in the medical journal, *Pediatrics*.

Walking the Baby Beat

This study was prompted by the case of a four-year-old boy in Souix Falls, South Dakota. He sustained a life-threatening perforation of the small intestine, very much like the child you describe.

The child's parents reported that his injury was caused by a fall down the stairs, which is a common explanation given by abusive parents to account for their children's injuries. Lacking absolute medical certainty to refute the parents' story, the doctors involved decided to do a study.

They searched all the medical articles written in English and published since 1970 for reports of injuries sustained in falls on stairs and for reports of small intestine perforations. Here's what they found:

- Of 312 cases of small intestinal perforation (65 in children), none were caused by falls on stairs.
- Of 677 cases of unobstructed falls on stairs (432 in children), none caused a small intestinal injury.
- Of the 65 cases of small intestinal perforation involving children, one-third was caused by motor vehicle accidents and one-third by physical assaults or child abuse.
- Of the 432 falls on stairs involving children, 69 percent sustained injuries of the head and neck and 22 percent sustained injuries of the arms or legs.

The researchers concluded that they found no evidence to suggest that an unobstructed fall on stairs could plausibly explain perforation of the small intestine. They went on to state that small intestine perforations combined with a delay in seeking medical care are a lethal form of child abuse.

This study explains why the doctors treating your friend's child suspected child abuse. It also suggests that your friend's child may still be in danger. What do you think?

D. Gary Benfield, M.D.

Cerebral palsy

DO INFANTS OUTGROW CEREBRAL PALSY?

Q *Our nine-month-old son was recently diagnosed with cerebral palsy. His doctor said it was a mild case, and he might outgrow it. Is that true? Do children outgrow cerebral palsy?*

A Children diagnosed at your son's age with mild cerebral palsy or CP often do "outgrow" their problem. In a large study of one-year-olds diagnosed with all types of CP, from mild to severe, about half were normal six years later. More relevant to your situation, three-fourths of those children initially diagnosed with mild CP at one year of age were later found to be normal.

You can help your son achieve his best by signing him up for an early intervention program, if you haven't done so already.

DOES HYPERBARIC OXYGEN HELP CEREBRAL PALSY?

Q *I recently read about a two-year-old boy in Brunswick, Ohio, who cannot sit, walk, or crawl without help. He has cerebral palsy. His parents are trying to raise $5,000 to fly him to England for treatments in a hyperbaric chamber. Does this treatment work? If it does, why isn't it offered in the United States?*

A When babies suffer brain damage before or at the time of birth, it can cause muscle tightness in the arms or legs or both. This muscle tightness leads to difficulty sitting, crawling, walking, and eating, depending on where the damage is located and how severe it is. This condition is known as cerebral palsy.

Walking the Baby Beat

In some instances, these children also have seizures and are mentally retarded. However, many have normal or above normal intelligence and do not have seizures.

A hyperbaric chamber is large enough to hold a patient and a medical team. The pressure in the chamber is increased above atmospheric pressure in order to increase the amount of oxygen in the inspired air.

This raises the amount of oxygen in the patient's bloodstream which, in turn, increases the amount of oxygen available to the tissues, including the brain.

Hyperbaric oxygen therapy has been used to treat the following conditions:

- Gas gangrene
- Carbon monoxide poisoning
- Deep sea divers who suffer from the bends, a painful condition that develops when a diver ascends too rapidly after being exposed to increased pressure under water.

Cerebral palsy results from *permanent damage* to a particular area of the brain. Therefore, supplying extra oxygen to the damaged area years later would seem like an exercise in futility.

In fact, too much oxygen may cause the arteries carrying blood to the brain to constrict, resulting in less than normal amounts of oxygen getting to the brain. This reaction may damage the normal surrounding brain and worsen the child's already compromised condition.

For all of these reasons, this therapy is not offered in the United States.

Until extensive studies of hyperbaric oxygen in animal models of cerebral palsy conclusively show a benefit, and those studies are replicated in humans, parents should think long and hard before they risk their child's health, their hard-earned money, and further disappointment on this kind of experiment.

D. Gary Benfield, M.D.

Sun protection

WHAT DOES THE SPF ON SUNSCREEN LOTIONS MEAN?

Q *Can you tell me what SPF stands for on a bottle of sunscreen lotion?*

A SPF stands for *sun protection factor,* the ratio of time it takes for the skin to burn with sunscreen on the skin to the time it takes to burn without sunscreen protection.

An SPF of 15, for example, means a person using sunscreen protection can spend 15 times longer in the sun without burning compared to a person without sunscreen protection.

A further thought: The lifetime risk of skin cancer can be reduced by almost 80 percent if a sunscreen with SPF 15 or higher is used regularly during the first 18 years of life.

PROTECTING CHILDREN FROM THE SUN

Q *We have three boys, ages 6 years, 4 years, and 10 months. On warm, sunny days, the two older boys love playing outside without a shirt on while I take the baby along and watch. But I worry about them getting too much sun while they're young and getting skin cancer later on. My husband says I worry too much and that skin cancer only comes from too much sun exposure later in life, not while you're young. Can you tell me who is right? Also, how should I dress the baby when we go outside on sunny days?*

A Warm, sunny days are wonderful, for young and old alike. But let's not get too carried away by allowing your sons to play shirtless in the sun, apparently without using sunscreen. Here's why:

- Between 60 and 80 percent of lifetime sun exposure occurs before we turn 18. That's because children spend more time outdoors than most adults, especially in the summer.
- The sun is the main cause of skin cancer, the most common form of cancer in the United States. In fact, a million new cases are diagnosed each year, which amounts to 2,700 new cases daily.
- Skin cancer does occur in children and young adults, but most people who get skin cancer are older. So your husband is right on that point, but not because of sun exposure later in life.
- Older people get skin cancer because they have already received too much of the sun's damaging rays when they were young. That's because our skin "remembers" each sunburn and each suntan, year after year, as far back as early childhood and adolescence. So you're right on that point.

Studies show that two or more blistering sunburns as a child or teen increase the risk of developing skin cancer later in life. So it's very important to protect babies and children from sunburn for two reasons:

- To prevent skin cancer in later years.
- To prevent the child from becoming seriously ill right now.

Many parents incorrectly assume the sun is dangerous only when it's shining brightly. In fact, it's the invisible ultraviolet rays, not the visible light rays that are most harmful. Your children actually may be exposed to more ultraviolet rays on foggy or hazy days, because they'll stay outside for a longer time. Here are four suggestions to help prevent sunburn:

- Try to minimize sun exposure when the peak ultraviolet rays occur, between 10 A.M. and 4 P.M.
- Always use sunscreen with a sun protection factor (SPF) of at least 15. Remember to apply the sunscreen half an hour before going out.
- Dress your infant son, and your older children, in lightweight cotton clothing with long sleeves and long pants.
- Keep your infant son in the shade as much as possible, and have him wear a wide-brimmed hat.

The signs of sunburn usually appear six to twelve hours after exposure, with the greatest discomfort during the first 24 hours.

If your child's burn is just red, warm, and uncomfortable, you can treat it yourself. Apply cool compresses to the burned areas or bathe in cool water. It's okay to give acetaminophen to help relieve pain.

However, if the sunburn causes blisters, fever, chills, headache, or a general feeling of malaise, call your doctor. Severe sunburn is dangerous and may require hospitalization.

DOES AN AFRICAN-AMERICAN BABY NEED SUN PROTECTION?

Q *My husband and I are black. Three weeks ago, we became the proud parents of our first child. When we take her outside, does she need the same protection from the sun as white babies do?*

A Yes. Some folks have the misconception that black skin needs no sun protection because it doesn't tan or burn. That's not true. All skin is capable of burning—especially baby skin—and needs protection from the sun. It means taking the same precautions as those listed in the preceding question and answer.

WHAT IS ADEQUATE SUN PROTECTION?

Q *Can you settle a friendly disagreement between my husband and me? He says our five-year-old daughter will be protected from the sun if she wears a baseball cap and an oversized white T-shirt that covers most of her body. I say she still needs sun screen no matter what she wears.*

A I'm with you. A baseball cap does not protect most of the face or any of the neck from the sun. A white T-shirt offers limited protection—it only has a sun protection factor (SPF) of 5. Your daughter still needs sunscreen with a SPF of 15 or higher.

Autism

WHERE CAN WE FIND RELIABLE INFORMATION ABOUT AUTISM?

Q *Finally, after almost two years of grappling with an often out-of-control child, our pediatrician says our two-year-old son is autistic. Unfortunately, the doctor is a man of few words. Can you tell me where we can find reliable information about this problem?*

A The best place to start is to contact the Autism Society of America (www.autism-society.org or call 1-800-328-8476). There you will find a helpful staff armed with lots of helpful information. ASA also has chapters in nearly every state where you can go for information, support, and encouragement. You can find their locations listed on the Web site.

Loss of a child

REMEMBERING OUR DECEASED CHILDREN

To be honest, I don't go to church very often. You see, I'm one of those people who believes God is everywhere. For instance, when I place my stethoscope on a baby's chest and hear the lub-dub, lub-dub of her beating heart, I believe that's God's voice speaking.

So it was a bit out of character when I walked up the steps to the First Congregational Church of Akron one December night for the Annual Remembrance Service, sponsored by Akron Children's Hospital.

Like so many others gathered there, I'd been busy all day, rushing around doing my job and even sneaking in a little Christmas shopping. Now, here I sat among hundreds of families who had lost a child. Some had lost two or even three. And some of them had been my patients.

The minister began the service by giving thanks for the gifts that had been placed at the altar by dozens of parents in memory of their deceased children. The gifts would be distributed to needy children just in time for Christmas.

Next, we stood and sang "Silent Night." By the time we reached the last phrase, "Sleep in heavenly peace," I had already dug into my box of Kleenex, one of hundreds that had been placed throughout the sanctuary.

Two nurses from Akron Children's then took turns reading off the list of names of the deceased children. A bell was rung from the back balcony after each name was read. They started with "We remember Natalie Allen" and ended, twenty minutes later, with "We remember Lauren Yacovazzi."

Each year, a parent is asked to speak about his or her own personal journey since the loss of their child. This year, Jane Nichols, who founded the bereavement program at Akron Children's, was the guest speaker.

Jane began by telling how, more than 30 years ago, she had lost a baby to congenital heart disease, which was not diagnosed until autopsy. Today, her baby's heart problem would, most likely, be diagnosed before birth and corrected with surgery.

Jane also spoke about a second baby's death. Only this time her baby was stillborn, the victim of a cord accident. At the time, she recalled, she had more questions than answers. She could find no support groups for bereaved parents and no books to help with her grief. At the time, she wondered, "Why me? Haven't I already paid my dues?"

In 1978, Jane's journey brought her to Akron Children's, where she started a new service to help parents of dying and newly deceased babies in the neonatal intensive care unit. Later, her job expanded to include the whole hospital.

Out of her own personal losses, Jane's mission in life turned out to be helping parents understand their grief and finding the strength to move on. She touched thousands of lives during a distinguished career.

Jane then announced she was retiring at the end of the year. And when she finished and was about to sit down, the audience gave her a standing ovation.

The woman sitting next to me said without Jane, she wouldn't have made it. Her teenage son had died earlier that year from an auto accident. By now, my box of Kleenex was empty.

The service ended with the lighting of the candles. A single candle was lighted at the end of the first row, down front. Then that person lighted the candle of the person standing next to her and so on, until the darkened sanctuary glowed with light.

We stood for a few moments with our heads bowed, as if gathering strength from the warmth that filled the room.

Then we filed out and headed for the meeting room, where we renewed old acquaintances and shared memories from the past, over punch and cookies.

Yes, it did me good to sit and weep with those wonderful families as we heard the names of their deceased children read aloud once again.

WHY IS THE NEWBORN AUTOPSY SO IMPORTANT?

Q *My sister's two-day-old baby recently died in intensive care. When the doctor asked about an autopsy, my sister asked me what I thought. I told her if it were my baby, I would say no. But she and her husband decided to go ahead. Was I wrong in thinking this way? Why is an autopsy so important when the parents are grieving so hard?*

A Sometimes, life isn't fair. And one of those times is when parents are told something is wrong with their baby, and then their baby dies.

One of the toughest things a doctor must do is to sit down with that family and break the bad news. The second most difficult thing a doctor must do is to discuss whether to perform an autopsy on their newly deceased baby. To some parents and close relatives it may seem cruel. A baby has just died, and you want to talk about an autopsy?

Personally, when I'm the doctor in that situation, I wait until after the parents have held their newly deceased baby and said their goodbyes. This may take several minutes or several hours. Then, I raise the question, "Where do we go from here?"

Because most parents don't quite know what to expect, they usually welcome my suggestions. I explain why an autopsy might be important. I suggest how they might go about making funeral arrangements. And I suggest how they might go about breaking the news to their extended family.

In several ways, the newborn autopsy is more important than one performed on an adult (unless, of course, the adult has died under unusual circumstances).

- The main reason for the newborn autopsy is to fully explain why this baby died. At such times, both parents, but especially the mother, often feel they are somehow to blame for their baby's death. The autopsy helps set the record straight.
- Studies show that even when a major birth defect has been detected before birth, up to 35 percent of these babies will have additional, unrecognized defects. When the autopsy does reveal a hidden defect or a genetic disorder, parents can use that information to plan for future pregnancies. Sharing this information with the extended family may help them plan too.
- The newborn autopsy also acts as a form of quality control. For example, procedures done on the baby or the act of birth itself may cause internal bleeding or other complications that may go undetected unless an autopsy is done. This kind of information helps hospitals and doctors monitor patient care and detect potentially unsafe practices, something we all want them to do.
- Finally, the newborn autopsy helps doctors learn so we can help other babies. It is one of the important ways progress is made in all of medicine.

A further thought: When I ask parents for permission to do an autopsy, I also stress how important it is for us to get back together again, whenever they feel ready, to share what we learned from the autopsy and to discuss how they're adjusting to their loss.

If parents are still undecided, I suggest they take whatever additional time they need to make an informed decision. Go home and talk it over. Call me if you have more questions. I would rather them decide not to have an autopsy than leave them with the memory I had somehow tried to coerce them into having one.

TRYING AGAIN AFTER A NEWBORN DEATH

Q *It has taken my husband and me almost five years to get up the courage to try again after our first baby passed away minutes after birth. We received a copy of the autopsy report and a letter from the doctor that said the cause of death was Potter's syndrome. Can you explain what Potter's syndrome is and what the chances are of it happening again?*

A Potter's syndrome is a fatal condition that was first described by Dr. Edith Potter, one of the first pediatric pathologists. After performing several thousand newborn autopsies over many years, Potter described 20 cases in which the kidneys had failed to develop (absent kidneys) and the lungs were too small to support life. Let me explain.

The normally developing fetus usually starts to urinate around the ninth week of pregnancy. This fetal urine becomes the main source of amniotic fluid that surrounds the developing fetus, forming a protective cushion between the fetus and the inner wall of the uterus. (That's correct, the amniotic fluid is composed primarily of fetal urine.)

If the kidneys fail to develop normally, then urine is not produced. Because the cushioning effect of amniotic fluid against the fetal chest wall is crucial for normal lung growth and development, this lack of fluid results in lungs that are too small to support life.

Walking the Baby Beat

From the moment of birth, a baby with this fatal condition will have difficulty breathing. Even with aggressive treatment, death usually occurs within a few hours.

Potter's syndrome occurs once in every 3,000 births. Even though your chances are very good that it won't happen again, it has occurred more than once in a small number of families.

It's very important for you and your husband to arrange with your doctor to order an ultrasound evaluation of your kidneys. Why? Because in one series of babies who died from Potter's syndrome, 9 percent of first-degree relatives (mother, father, and siblings) were found to have kidney defects themselves that were not causing symptoms.

Also, before trying again, you and your husband should also talk with your doctor about referring you to a genetics counselor. When you go for your counseling appointment, be sure to take along a copy of the letter you received about your son's autopsy and a copy of his medical record.

A further thought: Since Dr. Potter first described Potter's syndrome, we've learned that some babies have kidneys filled with cysts that compromise their ability to produce adequate amounts of urine during pregnancy. As a result, they too are born with small lungs and breathing problems that are often, but not always, incompatible with life. With long-term life support, meaning months to years, combined with a kidney transplant, some of these babies have actually survived.

So now the definition of Potter's syndrome has expanded to include these babies too, creating a dilemma for some parents when their baby is born with Potter's syndrome. Should we forgo life support and let our baby die in peace, or should we put our baby through months to years of suffering with no guarantee of survival, much less a healthy outcome?

D. Gary Benfield, M.D.

WHEN A BABY DIES, FORGET THE FREE ADVICE

Q *Not so long ago, our baby passed away from an overwhelming infection. Perfectly formed in every way, our beautiful baby drew her last breath as my wife and I held her and cried.*

Everyone, including the doctors and nurses, were very kind and supportive. But toward the end of the graveside service, the minister turned to my wife and said, "Now God has a little angel in heaven. Remember, you are both young and can try again." My wife got so upset, she had to walk away.

Please tell your readers that when a couple has lost a baby, at least have the courtesy to forget the advice, and just be there with open arms.

A Thank you for the reminder. You've said it better than anything I can say.

SHOULD A CHILD BE ALLOWED TO TOUCH HER DECEASED BABY BROTHER?

Q *I would like your opinion about something that has bothered me ever since my sister's six-week-old baby died of SIDS.*

At calling hours, the baby lay in an open casket, dressed in a cute blue outfit complete with a bonnet and booties. His eyes were closed, and he looked like he was taking a nap.

As I stood nearby and watched, my sister's five-year-old daughter walked up to the casket and asked if she could touch her baby brother. My sister reached down and gently took her daughter's hand and touched it to the baby's cheek.

Do you think it's proper for a five-year-old to see, let alone touch, a dead baby? What purpose could it possibly serve?

A A death in the family should be shared by all members of the family. But children are often forgotten by grieving adults. When we overlook or forbid them from meeting their needs and surround them with silence and secrecy, we risk increasing their sense of isolation and adding to their confusion.

Not only was it appropriate for your niece to see and touch her newly deceased brother, your sister deserves your support for handling the situation in a straightforward and caring manner, in my opinion. Should children be shielded from death? Rarely, if ever.

A further thought: No matter how helpful calling hours or the funeral may be for some of us, children should not be forced to attend. If an apprehensive youngster prefers to remain at home, don't put pressure on her just to get your way. Perhaps the time will come later when the two of you might visit the cemetery together.

A NURSE PULLED THE CURTAIN BETWEEN THIS MOTHER AND HER DYING BABY

"And what do you do?" the saleswoman asked as I handed her my credit card. She wore a dark blue suit and a bright smile that forced me to smile in return. Her gold-plated name tag read, "Jennifer, 34 Years of Service."
 "I'm a neonatologist,"
 "A what?"
 "A neonatologist," I said. "I'm like a firefighter or a police officer. Folks don't want me around when things are going well. But if their baby has a problem, they're glad to see me."
 "Oh," she said. "You must work with those tiny babies in neonatal."

"Actually, about half of them are tiny," I said. "Full-term babies have problems too. Things like serious birth defects or life-threatening infections."

"Really?" she said. "That must be hard, especially when so many babies don't make it."

She handed me my card, and I signed the receipt. As I handed it back, I sensed something was wrong. Her eyes were moist, and her hand was shaking.

"I'm sorry," I said. "Sometimes I talk too much."

"It's not your fault," she said. "You have no way of knowing that we lost a baby almost 32 years ago."

"Would you like to tell me what happened?"

"I remember it like it was yesterday," she said. "He only lived for 12 hours. I was standing outside the nursery, watching through the glass, when he finally stopped breathing. A nurse pulled the curtain and that was it. I never saw him again. The doctor came to my room and said my baby had gotten infected as he passed through the birth canal. Then he turned and walked away. That's the way things were done in those days."

"I'm so sorry,"

"Actually, it does me good to talk about it," she said. "Not a day goes by that I don't think about him. But there's no one to talk to, not even my husband. His only son, you know."

"Did you try again after that?"

"We had two lovely girls after that," she said. "The oldest is married and works as a computer programmer. The youngest is in graduate school. We never told them about their brother."

"I'd like to hear more about what you and your husband went through," I said. "But I'm late for my daughter's birthday party. Perhaps we could arrange to talk some more, and you could teach me what it was like so I can help other parents. Who knows, you might learn something too."

"I'd like that very much," she said. "If we could meet at our house, I might convince my husband to join us."

"That's fine with me," I said. "Here's my card. Just call me when you're ready."

With that, the delightful, white-haired lady reached across the counter, took my hands in hers, and shook them warmly. "Thank you," she said.

I left the store wondering whether she would actually call. I thought she probably would, but I didn't know what to think about her husband.

Two weeks later, Jennifer and her husband, Tom, greeted me at their front door and invited me in. We sat down to coffee and cookies and talked for hours. Then, just as our conversation was drawing to a close, Tom suddenly opened up and told his side of the story.

For the past 32 years, not a day had passed that he, too, hadn't thought about their son. He had kept it bottled up, because he didn't want to upset his wife or their daughters.

As we stood at the door and said our goodbyes, I suggested they consider calling a family meeting. Their daughters should know they had a brother who lived for a short time, died from an infection, and was loved by their parents just as they had been too.

They looked at each other and both nodded yes.

A further thought: This story shows what can happen when a physician doesn't take the time to sit down with newly bereaved parents and discuss not only what caused their child's death, but answer all their questions and encourage them to share their feelings. It also shows what can happen when a parent's last memory of her baby is a nurse pulling the curtain between her and her dying child.

SHOULD PARENTS TALK ABOUT DEATH WITH THEIR DYING CHILD?

Talking to myself about the most difficult thing a parent may ever do: Talk about death with a dying child who has a malignant disease.

  I: So what do you think?
Me: About what?
  I: This issue.
Me: What issue?
  I: You know, the death issue.
Me: What death issue?
  I: The one nobody wants to talk about.
Me: What do you think I am, a mind reader? Spit it out.
  I: Do you think a parent should talk about death with a dying child who has a malignant disease?
Me: How do you know for sure the child is dying?
  I: There you go again, answering my question with a question.
Me: It's an important question.
  I: Why is that?
Me: Put yourself in the parents' shoes.
  I: Okay
Me: Their 14-year-old daughter, let's call her Amy, was diagnosed two years ago with a malignant brain tumor.
  I: Go on.
Me: For the past two years, Amy's doctors tried everything: radiation, surgery, perhaps even chemotherapy.
  I: Okay.
Me: During that time, Amy had mostly good days. Her parents took her to Disneyland, and she got to meet Mia Hamm, her favorite soccer player.
  I: Go on.

Me: But now, she's having more bad days than good days. She can't keep anything down. She's lost 15 pounds over the past month, and she's having difficulty seeing out of her left eye. She senses something is terribly wrong and that she may be dying.

I: So, what's your point?

Me: My point is Amy's parents won't let themselves believe their lovely Amy is dying. Even though Amy's doctor has brought it up, her parents are searching the Web constantly, leaving no stone unturned, trying to find a cure for their child. They don't want to hear the awful truth that Amy is dying. To them, that means they've failed her.

I: What happens next?

Me: If Amy's parents can't accept there is no cure, that Amy is truly dying, then Amy may die alone with her thoughts and fears, although she's surrounded by family and friends.

I: Wow!

Me: Wow is right. The tragedy is it's well known that kids in these kinds of situations sense they're dying. But many parents, in their quest for a cure, won't let themselves see what their child may need most: the opportunity to talk about death, the opportunity to be in tune in with her parents, the opportunity to be genuinely supported at the end.

I: So it's not so much a question of should Amy's parents talk with her about death, but, rather, how do we get them to accept that Amy is dying, that she might want to talk about death, and that they haven't failed her by bringing it up, right?

Me: Exactly. It just so happens a recent study from Sweden deals precisely with your question.

I: What did the study find?

Me: Researchers contacted all the parents in Sweden who had lost a child to cancer between 1992 and

D. Gary Benfield, M.D.

1997. None of the 147 parents who had talked with their child about death regretted it. But 27 percent of the 258 parents who hadn't talked to their child about death regretted not having done so.
I: A powerful message.
Me: No doubt about it.

School health

NIT-PICKING ABOUT HEAD LICE

Talking to myself about head lice in children:

I: You're writing about head lice?
Me: That's right.
I: Just the thought makes me cringe.
Me: Cringe?
I: You know, makes me itchy.
Me: Can I tell you why I'm writing about head lice?
I: Be my guest.
Me: The main reason is most parents of school-aged children and many school administrators don't understand the problem. Head lice are not a health hazard or a lack of cleanliness. All they do is cause itching.
I: Are you saying it's no big deal?
Me: Not exactly. What I am saying is head lice embarrasses kids and causes them to miss too much school. Head lice also embarrasses their parents and causes them to miss time from work.
I: How come you're so smart, all of a sudden?
Me: I recently read the American Academy of Pediatrics' policy on head lice.
I: Does the policy say kids with head lice should stay in school?

Walking the Baby Beat

Me: No. But it does say a child should be allowed to return to school the next day after proper treatment.
I: What's proper treatment?
Me: The Academy recommends a product called NIX, a cream rinse that is applied to the hair after the hair has been shampooed with a non-conditioning shampoo and towel dried. NIX is left on for 10 minutes and then rinsed off, leaving a residue on the hair to kill any remaining eggs or nits. One treatment is usually enough, but sometimes a second treatment is necessary, if live lice are seen 7–10 days later.
I: That's it?
Me: There's more. The child's hair should be combed with a fine-tooth comb to remove the dead eggs and any nits that may have survived treatment. To prevent reinfection, parents should also wash all bedclothes and clothing (hats are a big culprit) that have been in contact with the child up to 48 hours before treatment. Combs and brushes can be soaked in very hot water. Other family members may also need to be treated and have their clothing and bedding laundered.
I: If the AAP recommends that a child with head lice be allowed to return to school the next day after treatment, why is so much time lost from school?
Me: Mainly because many schools have a "no-nit" policy. So, if even one dead nit remains, the child is not allowed to return to school until her hair is nit-free. A second reason is that almost 50 percent of the time head lice is misdiagnosed, leading to unnecessary treatment and loss of time from school.
I: Does the AAP say anything about this no-nit policy?
Me: The AAP discourages no-nit policies for returning to school.
I: I'll bet it's an emotional issue for parents.
Me: Didn't you say it makes you itchy?

I: I have to admit you helped me get over that. Maybe it would help others if they could read the AAP's new policy for themselves.

Me: That's a good idea. It's on the AAP's Web site, www.aap.org. Type "no nit policy" in the Search box and click on "New Head Lice Statement: AAP Discourages 'No Nit' Policies for School Return," and print it out.

A further thought: Several readers asked for more details about head lice, so here goes:

Head lice come in three forms:

- The nit
- The nymph
- The adult louse

Nits are lice eggs. They are hard to see and easily confused with dandruff or hair spray droplets. However, nits are firmly attached to the hair shaft; dandruff and hair spray are not.

The nit hatches into a baby louse or nymph. It looks like an adult louse but is smaller. Nymphs mature into adults about 9–12 days after hatching.

The adult louse is about the size of a sesame seed, has six legs, and is tan to grayish-white. The female louse lives for three to four weeks. After mating, she lays about 10 eggs, or nits, per day. The tiny eggs are firmly attached to the hair shaft, close to the scalp, with a glue-like substance produced by the louse.

The eggs are incubated by scalp heat and hatch in 10–14 days. Once the eggs hatch, nymphs leave the shell covering, grow for about 9–12 days, and then, after mating, the females lay eggs. If untreated, this cycle repeats itself every three weeks.

The louse ejects small amounts of saliva onto the scalp then feeds by removing tiny amounts of blood from the scalp every few hours. The saliva creates an itchy irritation. But itching is often delayed for four to six weeks, the time it takes for sensitivity to louse saliva to develop.

Head lice cannot hop or fly; they crawl. Transmission from person to person commonly occurs by head-to-head contact. Because head lice normally survive for less than 24 hours away from the scalp at room temperature, and because their eggs cannot hatch at a temperature lower than that of the scalp, indirect spread by contact with an infested person's personal items is uncommon, but does occur. Thus, it's prudent to teach children not to share personal items such as head combs, brushes, and hats.

The gold standard for diagnosing head lice is to find and capture a live louse on the head. Nits are easiest to spot along the nape of the neck or behind the ears, just inside the hairline.

It's probably impossible to totally prevent head lice infestations because young children often come into close head-to-head contact. Manual removal of nits after treatment is only necessary for aesthetic reasons or to decrease diagnostic confusion.

The recommended treatment is 1 percent permethrin (brand name NIX) applied as a 10-minute rinse. One treatment is usually enough. A child should be allowed to return to school the next day after treatment.

However, some schools have no-nit policies that forbid returning to school until all nits are removed. The American Academy of Pediatrics (www.aap.org) and the National Association of School Nurses (www.nasn.org) discourage such policies. They believe that children with head lice should not be excluded from school, once they have been adequately treated.

In the United States, head lice are less common in African-American children than in children of other races, probably because African-Americans have oval-shaped hair shafts that are harder for lice to grasp. In Africa, however, head lice have adapted claws for grasping this type of hair.

D. Gary Benfield, M.D.

Teen health concerns

CHILDREN WITH DIABETES CAN PLAY ANY SPORT IF . . .

Q *Our daughter will be in the ninth grade this fall and is dead set on trying out for the volleyball team. The problem is she takes insulin for diabetes, and she was born with one ovary. Can you tell us whether it's safe for her to play?*

A Children with diabetes can play any sport if they do the following:

- Pay attention to their diet.
- Stay well hydrated.
- Monitor their glucose level.
- Adjust their insulin dose accordingly.

The risk of injury to your daughter's ovary is minimal and should not prevent her from competing.

Why don't you consider going with your daughter to discuss her plans with her doctor. If her doctor agrees that it's safe for her to play, ask if he would mind writing a note for the school principal, stating that in his medical opinion it's safe for her to play. Then you and your daughter should schedule a meeting with the school principal to present the note and make sure he knows and agrees that she's cleared to play.

It's important to avoid the temptation to run interference for your daughter and do all of this yourself. Don't fall into that trap. By involving her every step along the way, you will help her learn how to manage her own health care. This skill is important for all teens, but especially if they have a chronic disease such as diabetes.

A further thought: While on the subject of medical conditions that might affect a child's ability to participate in sports, parents need to remember that children who have a fever should not compete until their temperature returns to normal. A fever does the following:

- Makes the heart and lungs work harder
- Reduces the capacity for exercise
- Increases the risk of heat-related illness

For more information, try the American Academy of Pediatrics web site (www.aap.org), look under policy statements, and click on "Medical Conditions Affecting Sports Participation."

WHEN A TUBAL PREGNANCY MIMICS APPENDICITIS

Q *My cousin's 15-year-old daughter was recently rushed to the hospital with a diagnosis of appendicitis. But when the doctor took her to surgery, he found a tubal pregnancy, not appendicitis. Can you explain how a tubal pregnancy can be mistaken for appendicitis?*

A In a female of child-bearing age, appendicitis and a tubal pregnancy can both present with the following symptoms:

- Abdominal pain
- Low-grade fever
- Nausea and vomiting

The findings on physical exam are also quite similar. The way to tell the difference between the two is to take a thorough history and order a pregnancy test.

Of course, a 15-year-old may deny being sexually active when she really is, which is why the pregnancy test is so useful; it doesn't lie. But a positive pregnancy test only confirms that the patient is pregnant. She may still have appendicitis and be pregnant at the same time. After all, appendicitis is the most common, acute, surgical emergency of pregnancy, affecting one in 2,000 pregnant women.

An ultrasound of the abdomen may come in handy at this point. An ultrasound that reveals a developing baby within the uterus rules out a tubal pregnancy. Conversely, if a baby cannot be visualized in the uterus, then a tubal pregnancy is more likely.

The information you've provided doesn't say whether a pregnancy test or an ultrasound was done. However, appendicitis and a tubal pregnancy are both life-threatening conditions, and both need surgical intervention as soon as possible.

SHOULD WE LET OUR SON GO FOR BEACH WEEK?

Q *Our son graduates from high school at the end of May. He and two of his senior buddies are planning a trip the following week to the beach at Ocean City, Maryland. They're good kids and paying their own way with money they've earned from working part-time jobs.*

The problem is we know these boys will be around a lot of drinking and probably drink themselves. My husband feels we should let him go, but I'm not so sure. Can you help us sort out what to do?

A For many high school seniors, "beach week" has become as much a part of graduation as the senior prom. Whether the beach is located along the East Coast, the West Coast, or south of the border in Mexico, beach week offers a lot more than the chance to relax on a sandy beach and throw down a few cold ones.

Some teens stay drunk and use marijuana daily. And while drunk, they often engage in sex. Some return home sporting a new tattoo or body piercing. Let's face it. The temptations are enough to make parents cringe.

On the other hand, beach week is a right of passage. For most graduates, it marks the first time they have been on their own. And although they will encounter many temptations, it's a time for teens to test their wings, to be faced with choices, and to accept the consequences of their actions.

Not all of these teens will drink, do drugs, or have sex. In fact, studies show that a teen's conduct during beach week is strongly related to his or her conduct at home.

So, it seems, the question boils down to this: If you trust your son's judgment at home and respect his desire for independence, can you trust his judgment while away from home in such a risky environment?

Perhaps you and your husband should sit down with your son and discuss this question. Deep down inside, I think you know the answer.

A further thought: Ocean City, Maryland, is a beach resort of some 15,000 permanent residents. In a typical summer, the city's population swells to 300,000 as thousands of "June bugs"—the city's nickname for high school graduates—flock there to celebrate.

Community residents welcome the young visitors but make it clear that underage drinking and the use of illicit drugs are no longer tolerated. Beverage servers and liquor stores are trained to detect fraudulent age documents and to turn away underage drinkers.

Meanwhile, police officers, in uniform and plain clothes, maintain a strong presence throughout the city. A citation brings a mandatory court appearance—a strong deterrent.

TEEN HEALTH AND THE LAW

Q *I'm 14 and want to get a prescription for the pill. Do I need my parents' consent?*

A No. Prescription contraceptives, like all other forms of contraception, are available to minors without parental consent. However, if you don't tell your parents and get their consent, you will have to pay for the pill yourself. Perhaps your doctor can help you talk to your parents or help you find low-cost or free pills.

A further thought: Another version of the above question goes something like this: My 16-year-old friend has gonorrhea and needs treatment, but she doesn't want to tell her parents she has a sexually transmitted disease. Can she get treated without her parent's consent? In general, the answer is "yes." But, once again, she'll have to pay for the treatment herself.

SHOULD TEENS BE INCLUDED IN DISCUSSIONS ABOUT THEIR HEALTH?

Q *I'm 13 and overweight. Every time my mom takes me to the doctor, they go into another room and talk. Then on the way home, she tells me what the doctor said. I don't think that's fair. Do you?*

A I'm on your side. You should be included (actually, "must" is a better word) in any discussion about your health when you and your mother go to the doctor. Then the doctor can talk to you directly, and you can ask questions. It's called taking responsibility for your own health.

Talk it over with your mom and your doctor. They may not realize how much leaving the room to talk bothers you.

WHAT IS AN EMANCIPATED MINOR?

Q *What is an emancipated minor? Is a minor who has given birth to a child considered emancipated?*

A A minor is considered emancipated when the parents no longer have control over the child. This can occur under the following circumstances:

- When a teen marries
- When a teen enlists in the armed services
- When a teen is incarcerated
- When a teen leaves home and can provide for him- or herself

A minor who has given birth to a child may be considered emancipated. She may be able to consent to her own health care and the health care for her child, but, according to the American Civil Liberties Union, no definite rule of law guides this situation.

If she doesn't have health insurance, a hospital or doctor may ask the minor parent how she is going to pay for treatment. If necessary, the situation may require getting the parents of the minor parent to consent and help pay for her medical care.

A further thought: From tattoos on their backs to belly and tongue piercings, many teens are adding art to their bodies. Like any surgical procedure, tattoos and piercing carry a risk of serious infection. Teens must therefore choose carefully the tattoo or piercing procedures they undergo.

In Ohio, the law requires parental consent before a minor can get a tattoo, a body piercing, or even an ear piercing with an ear-piercing gun. A parent must go with the child to the place where the procedure will be performed and sign a document that describes the tattoo or piercing procedure and explains how to take care of the affected area after the procedure.

The law forbids a minor from lying about her age or forging her parent's signature. It's also illegal for a person to impersonate a minor's parent in order to help the minor obtain a tattoo or body piercing.

IS MY 13-YEAR-OLD'S BLOOD PRESSURE NORMAL?

Q *Our 13-year-old son recently came down with a bad cold. We treated him for several days with a decongestant, "Tylenol Sinus," and kept him home from school. When he didn't improve, I took him to our family doctor who prescribed an antibiotic and said to return in two weeks, which we did.*

The office nurse said my son's blood pressure was high at the first visit but normal at the second. The doctor said our son was probably anxious during the first visit, and that can sometimes raise the pressure. They also used a different blood pressure cuff for the second measurement, which he said gave a more accurate reading. Does his explanation sound right to you? Can you tell me whether our son's blood pressure is normal?

A Not knowing the actual readings makes it difficult to answer your question. However, your doctor was wise in having your son return for follow up and a second blood pressure reading.

The anxiety your doctor referred to is commonly known as the "white coat" effect. The blood pressure of certain people goes up when it's measured in the doctor's office. But when it's measured at home, under more relaxed conditions, the reading is often normal.

It also sounds like the first measurement was taken with a blood pressure cuff that was too narrow for your son's arm. This factor can yield an elevated reading.

The third factor that may have contributed to your son's elevated blood pressure is the decongestant your son was taking for his upper respiratory infection. Pseudoephedrine, the active ingredient in Tylenol Sinus and many other decongestants, can raise a person's blood pressure.

Fortunately, the blood pressure reverts to normal when the medication is stopped.

It sounds like your son's blood pressure is probably normal. However, if you are still concerned, you may want to have it rechecked periodically in a nonthreatening environment.

A further thought: Compared to adults, high blood pressure or hypertension occurs uncommonly in children and adolescents.

The two types of hypertension are primary and secondary. Primary hypertension—meaning we don't know the cause—accounts for 15 to 30 percent of all cases in adolescents. Thus 70 to 85 percent of hypertensive adolescents fall into the secondary category—meaning a cause can be identified if you search hard enough. Various kidney ailments top the list, followed by congenital heart defects, endocrine disorders, and tumors.

To avoid overdiagnosing high blood pressure in children, it's important to remember the following:

- A child's blood pressure normally increases with age.
- Normal values differ slightly for boys and for girls.
- At least three abnormal readings, obtained on separate occasions, should be obtained before making the diagnosis of hypertension in a child. This may require taking several readings at home or at school to avoid the "white coat" effect.

GONORRHEA IN TEENS: A SNEAKY, OFTEN SILENT DISEASE

Q *I'm worried and hope you can help me. My boyfriend and I are both high school seniors. He stopped me in the hall yesterday and said his family doctor has started him on antibiotics for gonorrhea. Then, he rushed off to baseball practice before I could ask any questions.*

D. Gary Benfield, M.D.

He and I have had sexual relations several times since we started going steady. I don't feel sick or anything. Should I take antibiotics too?

A You should see your doctor as soon as possible. (Preferably, you should take a parent along, but that's up to you.) After the doctor takes a history and examines you, he will probably do some tests. Then he will tell you whether you have the disease and need antibiotics.

Gonorrhea is a highly contagious, sexually transmitted disease. About 400,000 cases are reported annually in this country. However, hundreds of thousands more Americans may have the disease and not know it.

The first symptoms of gonorrhea may not appear for one to three weeks after sexual contact, if at all. Symptoms are often so mild you may not realize you have an infection. Frequently, the only clue that you have gonorrhea occurs when someone else who has had sexual contact with you develops the disease.

Early on, gonorrhea usually attacks a woman's cervix and urethra. That's why many women experience frequent, urgent, and painful urination along with an abnormal discharge from the vagina or urethra. However, in about half the cases, the only symptom is a slight increase in vaginal discharge.

If a woman has gonorrhea and doesn't receive early treatment, one or more of the following complications can occur:

- **Pelvic inflammatory disease.** The bacteria can spread into the uterus and out into the uterine tubes, causing pelvic inflammatory disease, or PID. PID is a serious infection that requires immediate treatment. Even with treatment, it frequently leaves behind scarred uterine tubes, a greater risk of ectopic or tubal pregnancy, and infertility. Between

10 and 40 percent of women infected with gonorrhea develop PID.
- **Conjunctivitis.** If the infection spreads to the eye by touching, it can cause a red, inflamed eye. In babies who contact gonorrhea during childbirth, untreated gonorrheal eye infection can lead to blindness.
- **Widespread infection.** The bacterium that causes gonorrhea can invade the bloodstream and cause infection in other parts of the body. Fever, rash, and joint pain are possible results.

Gonorrhea spreads through unprotected sexual contact—heterosexual or homosexual—with an infected partner. The more sexual partners you have, the greater your risk.

Teenagers have higher rates of gonorrhea than any other age group.

A further thought: This information is probably more than you may care to know about this sneaky, often silent disease. But it's important for all women to have this information because a case of gonorrhea may lead to PID, which can scar the uterine tubes and prevent a woman from ever having children. Similarly, in men, gonorrhea can cause inflammation of the testicles, which can also lead to infertility and an inability to have children. Scary thoughts? Yes.

DISCUSSING PREGNANCY PREVENTION WITH TEENS

Q *I recently had a frank discussion about sex with our 15-year-old daughter. But when our conversation turned to contraception, she asked a question I couldn't answer. Can you tell us the most effective way to keep from getting pregnant?*

D. Gary Benfield, M.D.

A The most effective way to keep from getting pregnant is avoid sexual intercourse. But since you were talking about contraception, I suspect you really meant to ask what's the most effective form of contraception to keep from getting pregnant? Before tackling that issue, let's say a bit more about abstinence.

- Abstinence is normal, common, and acceptable; we can show our affection in other ways besides having sex.
- Abstinence should be suggested and encouraged, stressing it as the best way to avoid pregnancy and to prevent sexually transmitted diseases (STDs).

It's also important to discuss the following with your daughter:

- Safe sexual behavior (holding hands, kissing, and fondling)
- Avoiding high-risk situations (using drugs and drinking)
- Practicing how to say no to sexual advances
- Encouraging her to discuss with partners what sexual activity is off limits

Many types of contraceptives are available. Here's a list of their success rates:

- Depo-Provera and Norplant, 99.6%
- Intrauterine device (IUD), 99.4%
- Oral contraceptive pills, 97%
- Condom, 88%
- Diaphragm, 82%
- Vaginal foam, 79%

Condoms should always be used in addition to other methods because, correctly used, condoms increase effectiveness and offer significant protection from STDs.

Millions of American teenagers are sexually active and need effective contraception. A discussion of pregnancy prevention methods, including abstinence, should be part of the doctor's visit for all adolescents.

Concern over the side effects of each method should be carefully discussed. However, it should be remembered that the risks of contraceptives are almost always far lower than the risks of pregnancy and childbirth.

A careful matching of the sexually active adolescent with an appropriate contraceptive method will help keep side effects to a minimum and increase compliance.

Because of continuing concerns about pelvic inflammatory disease (infection involving the uterine tubes) related to using IUDs, these devices are not recommended for most adolescents.

A further thought: A discussion of pregnancy prevention methods, including abstinence, as well as the other topics mentioned, should be part of every high school curriculum. However, not everyone agrees with this statement.

KEYS TO LIFELONG BONE HEALTH

Q *Our daughter is an very active 13 year-old who plays tennis almost daily. Can you tell me how much calcium she needs in her diet to have strong, healthy bones?*

A Before answering your question, it's important to remember that strong, healthy bones require an adequate intake of calcium *and* vitamin D; the two work together. Consuming foods rich in calcium and vitamin D is a key to lifelong bone health. Another key, which your daughter is already doing, is regular exercise.

In 1997, the Institute of Medicine revised its guidelines for daily calcium and vitamin D intake for children and adolescents. These new guidelines take into account the tremendous gain in bone mass during the pubertal growth spurt.

To ensure an adequate supply of calcium during this period of rapid growth, the recommended dietary calcium intake was increased to 1,300 milligrams (mg) per day, starting at age 9 and continuing until the age of 18. Dairy products are the main source of daily calcium intake for most children. They can usually obtain adequate calcium and vitamin D from these sources, especially if vitamin D–fortified milk is part of the diet.

Each 8-ounce glass of milk contains about 300 mg of calcium, whether its whole milk, reduced fat, or nonfat milk. So three glasses of milk daily will provide 900 mg of your daughter's 1,300 mg daily requirement. Add a cup of calcium-fortified cereal, which contains 300 mg of calcium, and mix in several ounces of milk, and your daughter's daily calcium requirement is met.

This combination also meets her daily vitamin D requirement. Other foods that contain significant amounts of calcium include calcium-fortified orange juice, most cheeses, low fat yogurt, pizza, and ice cream.

Many vegetables, such as broccoli, contain substantial amounts of calcium, but the calcium in some vegetables is not easily absorbed. Spinach, for example, is relatively rich in calcium, but it's also high in oxalates that bind calcium, reducing calcium's availability. Thus, only about 5 percent of the calcium in spinach is actually absorbed.

Many nondairy products are now fortified with calcium and provide the same, or only slightly less, calcium as comparable servings of milk. Foods popular with adolescents, such as waffles, cereal bars, fruit juices, and some breads are fortified with calcium. These foods are useful sources of calcium for adolescents who don't like or cannot tolerate dairy products.

Aside from fortified dairy products and breakfast cereals, the main source of vitamin D is exposure to sunlight. Darkly pigmented skin decreases the production of vitamin D in response to sunlight. In fact, dark-skinned adolescents may need up to six times more light exposure than light-skinned children to synthesize the same amount of vitamin D. This means black children require more time in the sun than white children to meet their vitamin D needs.

A further thought: Families should remember that regular exercise is an important key to building strong bones. For many adolescents, it means spending less time browsing the Internet or watching TV and more time exercising.

ECSTACY IS NOTHING TO RAVE ABOUT

Talking to myself about the teen rave scene and Ecstasy:

I: Okay, Bubba, tell me about those parties where teenagers dance all night and get high on Ecstasy.
Me: You mean raves?
I: That's it.
Me: Raves are dumb and nothing but trouble.
I: Tell me what you really think.
Me: Raves last all night, right?
I: If you say so.
Me: So you need something to help you stay up all night and still feel connected to others, right?
I: Makes sense to me.
Me: That's where a stimulant like Ecstasy comes in. It also makes you feel sexy and uninhibited.
I: What's wrong with that?
Me: It's a banned substance, knucklehead.
I: Just because it helps people lighten up?
Me: No, because it's dangerous. Here, let me explain. Ecstasy revs up your whole body. Your heart races, your arteries constrict, and your blood pressure can shoot sky high. And if that isn't bad enough, your body temperature starts to climb, your teeth clench together, your vision gets blurred, and you

can get chills, the sweats, dry mouth, and have seizures. In one study, Ecstasy was the second leading cause of liver damage in people under 25.

I: Amazing!

Me: Wait, there's more. Cat scans have detected brain damage in recreational users up to seven years later.

I: Really?

Me: Really. You can also get confused, depressed, insomnia, drug cravings, anxious, and have feelings of paranoia which can last for weeks. Ecstasy has caused liver failure, cardiac arrest, strokes, heart attacks, hyperthermia, and suicide.

I: I had no idea.

Me: You and a lot of folks. Another reason Ecstasy is so dangerous is because you have no way of knowing how much drug you're getting.

I: How so?

Me: It's often cut with other drugs that have their own dangerous side effects.

I: Is it easy to find?

Me: In one survey, more than half of all high school students said it's easy to find. Experts say nearly 12 percent of high school seniors have tried it at least once.

I: Thanks for the education, Bubba.

Me: My pleasure, knucklehead.

I: One last question.

Me: Shoot.

I: Have you ever tried Ecstasy yourself?

Me: Are you kidding? I haven't even tried marijuana.

DOES OBESITY RUN IN FAMILIES?

Q *My daughter and her husband are both at least 50 pounds overweight and have been that way long before they were mar-*

ried. *They have three teenagers, ages 18, 15, and 13. All three are on the heavy side, but probably not more than 10 to 15 pounds overweight.*

Can you tell me whether obesity runs in families? If so, are these three grandchildren of mine more likely to grow up obese like their parents?

A It has long been recognized that obesity runs in families. For a child, if one parent is obese, the child is three times as likely to be an obese adult as a child whose parents are not obese. If both parents are obese, the child is 10 times more likely to grow up obese than a child whose parents are not obese.

A further thought: American children are growing fatter and fatter with each passing day. Currently, 15.5 percent of all 12- to 19-year-olds are classified as obese, according to the American Academy of Pediatrics.

For these children, the ratio of weight to the square of their height, known as the body mass index, exceeds that of 95 percent of kids their age.

In addition, more and more children younger than five are becoming overweight and obese.

As if those statistics aren't bad enough, children and adolescents today are less physically active as a group than were previous generations, and less active children are more likely to be overweight.

We all know that obesity is bad for you at any age. In the pediatric age group obesity is associated with the following conditions:

- Heart problems
- High blood pressure
- Type 2 diabetes
- Menstrual irregularity
- Depression
- Low self-esteem

Some experts believe that the psychological stress of being ostracized is just as damaging as these medical problems.

Not a pretty picture.

CHILDHOOD OBESITY AND DIABETES OFTEN GO HAND IN HAND

Q *My 15-year-old grandson was recently diagnosed with what the doctor calls type 2 diabetes. He said the diabetes was mainly caused by my grandson's weight problem. Can you explain how obesity leads to diabetes?*

A Let's start by explaining diabetes itself and reviewing the different types of diabetes. Then my answer will make more sense.

Diabetes is a disease in which blood sugar levels are higher than normal. Why? Because people with diabetes have a problem converting food to energy. Let me explain.

After we eat food, it's broken down into fat, protein, and glucose in our intestine, absorbed into our blood stream, and carried to cells throughout our bodies. In order for our cells to absorb glucose and convert it into energy, our cells need insulin, a hormone made by the pancreas.

People develop diabetes because the pancreas does not make enough insulin or because the cells in their bodies do not use the insulin properly, or both. Either way, the amount of glucose in their blood increases and their cells are starved of energy.

If the high blood glucose, also called hyperglycemia, persists, it damages nerves and blood vessels, leading to the following complications:

- Heart disease and stroke
- Kidney disease

- Blindness
- Nerve damage and circulation problems

The three types of diabetes are as follow:

- Type 1 diabetes was formerly called juvenile diabetes. That's because it used to be the only type of diabetes seen in children, teenagers, and young adults. In this form of diabetes, the islet cells of the pancreas, which produce insulin, no longer make adequate insulin because the body's immune system has attacked and destroyed them.
- Type 2 diabetes is the most common form of diabetes and used to be called adult-onset diabetes. Years ago, it was rarely diagnosed in children, teenagers, or young adults. This form of diabetes usually begins with insulin resistance, meaning the body's cells do not use insulin properly. At first, when this situation occurs, the pancreas compensates by producing more insulin. In time, however, the pancreas gets exhausted and loses its ability to secrete enough insulin to keep up with the demand created by meals.
- The third type of diabetes is called gestational diabetes, occurring in some women during pregnancy. This type of diabetes tends to resolve after the baby is born, but a woman who has developed gestational diabetes is more likely to develop type 2 diabetes later in life.

Now, let's return to your question: How does obesity lead to diabetes in children?

Normally, in response to a meal, the pancreas produces insulin, which acts on the cells in our bodies, enabling them to absorb glucose and convert it to energy. So far, so good. But in obese people, the cells gradually develop insulin resistance, meaning cells fail to respond to insulin.

Early in this sequence, the pancreas is able to keep up by producing more insulin, maintaining a normal blood glucose level. At a certain point, however, the pancreas fails to keep up, resulting in an elevated blood glucose level.

Early on, this process is silent, often evading detection until a parent notices that her child has developed one or more of the following symptoms:

- Frequent urination
- Increased thirst
- Unexplained weight loss

Other symptoms may include the following:

- Fatigue
- Blurred vision
- Increased hunger
- Sores that don't heal

Then someone gets suspicious and draws blood for a glucose level and finds it elevated.

A further thought: We are experiencing an epidemic of childhood obesity in this country. As a result, type 2 diabetes is striking more children than ever before. In fact, type 2 diabetes has even replaced type 1 diabetes as the most common form of childhood diabetes in some clinics.

IS OBESITY SURGERY A GOOD IDEA FOR TEENS?

Talking to myself about gastric bypass surgery for obese teenagers:

I: So what do you think about Amy Topel's surgery?
Me: Who's Amy Topel?

Walking the Baby Beat

I: She's the 15-year-old who made the news after gastric bypass surgery.
Me: How much did she weigh?
I: Two hundred and sixty pounds.
Me: A real fatty!
I: That's what her classmates called her.
Me: Sorry, Amy. I was just fooling around.
I: That's also what her classmates said.
Me: Okay, already. Get on with your story.
I: According to news reports, she'd tried everything—all kinds of diets, exercise, and even diet pills. Apparently, nothing worked.
Me: Who did her surgery?
I: A surgeon in Chicago. He also did the same procedure on Amy's mother awhile back.
Me: Really?
I: Really. They suffered from the same problem; they ate too much. Now, back to my question. What do you think about a 15-year-old undergoing this kind of surgery?
Me: It bothers me a lot.
I: How so, oh wise one?
Me: First off, the surgery has risks: wound infections, stomach leaks, and even blood clots.
I: But obesity also has risks: diabetes, heart disease, and high blood pressure, just to name a few.
Me: I'll grant you that. But not all teens are mature enough and have the family support to help them follow the rules after surgery.
I: What rules are you talking about?
Me: They have to eat smaller servings, count calories, make sure they get enough protein, and take extra vitamins, including calcium, to prevent bone loss. Some of these kids are used to gorging. But after they've had the surgery and their brain tells them to eat but their stomach says no, which one will they listen to?

I: Sounds like these kids could use psychological testing and some counseling to help predict which ones would have the best outcomes going in.
Me: That's right. If they go back to gorging, that causes vomiting. Then the body no longer processes sugar correctly leading to dizziness and diarrhea.
I: That's a gruesome thought.
Me: Some have not only gained back the weight, but there have been instances in which their smaller stomachs have ruptured from overeating.
I: What's your solution?
Me: I'm all for being cautious about lowering the age for this kind of surgery.
I: Where would you draw the line?
Me: I'd draw up new guidelines like some experts are doing now. The guidelines should insist on at least these three things: (1) Hospitals should pick a panel of experts to evaluate each teen's physical and emotional well-being and pick the best candidates. (2) Don't operate before teens have reached their full height potential, which is about age 13 for girls and 15 for boys. (3) Keep track of all patients until they're at least 21 so we can learn about unforeseen complications and side effects that may take years to develop.
I: Good start. Thank you.
Me: My pleasure.

WHEN A TEENAGER IS GENETICALLY DIFFERENT FROM HER PEERS

Many genetic disorders are not uncovered or even suspected until affected individuals reach adolescence or later. Then when the disorder is finally diagnosed, the news may turn a patient's life upside down.

Walking the Baby Beat

The following case history illustrates the difficulties a teenager may face when she realizes how different she is from her peers. The case also shows how she handles the news when the genetic cause is discovered.

Laurel Roach was a shy ninth grader. Not quite five feet tall, she had short blond hair, brown eyes, and a winning smile. A straight-A student, she had yet to miss a day of school. But since starting ninth grade, school was not as much fun as it used to be because now she had to take gym.

Laurel hated undressing and showering in front of the other girls. They had pubic hair and budding breasts, yet Laurel hadn't changed. She was so embarrassed by her shapeless, little-girl figure.

Laurel could sense the other girls staring at her and giggling behind her back. And, to make matters worse, it seemed like all of the girls in her class had started having their menstrual periods except her.

After the Thanksgiving holiday, even the boys in Laurel's class seemed to be making fun of her as they passed in the hall between classes. Before long, her smile faded, and her grades dropped.

Soon she was skipping school. When she hit rock bottom, Laurel gathered her courage, sat down with her parents, and poured out her tearful story.

They listened intently then held her close when she was done. After that, Laurel's parents made an appointment for her to see a specialist, who ordered some tests and discovered Laurel's problem.

The doctor said her lack of pubic hair and breast development, as well as her short stature and failure to menstruate, were all caused by a genetic disorder called Turner's syndrome, or TS.

Instead of having 46 chromosomes in every cell in her body, Laurel's cells only contained 45 chromosomes. She was missing one of her two sex chromosomes. And since 99 percent of women who conceive a baby with TS spontaneously miscarry, Laurel was lucky to be alive.

The doctor explained that all girls with TS are short, and more than 90 percent lack normal ovarian tissue. As a result, girls with TS don't produce the hormones necessary for pubic hair and breast tissue development. And because girls with TS don't ovulate, they don't have menstrual periods and can't become pregnant, at least not in the usual way.

TS patients frequently have other physical problems such as heart defects, kidney defects, hearing loss, and swelling of the hands and feet. Socially, girls with TS tend to be shy and withdrawn. Most have normal intelligence.

In addition to the complications resulting from their congenital anomalies, women with TS have an increased risk of osteoporosis, thyroiditis, diabetes, and inflammatory bowel disease.

At first, Laurel was devastated by the news. But when further tests showed her heart and kidneys were normal and that her hearing was not affected, she started to perk up. After all, I'm lucky to be alive, she said.

So, in step-wise fashion over the next three years, the doctor prescribed a course of growth hormone that added four inches to her height, started estrogen therapy to promote pubic hair and breast development, and added progesterone to induce her menstrual cycle.

By the time Laurel graduated from high school, she had regained her self-confidence and her love for school, and was looking forward to attending college.

And one more thing: She even dreamed that someday she might be able to have children using in vitro fertilization and ovum donation.

WHAT IS MEANT BY HEAT-RELATED ILLNESS?

Q *Can you explain what is meant by the term "heat-related illness"? Does it have something to do with heatstroke?*

A Heat-related illnesses include the following:

- Heat cramps
- Heat exhaustion
- Heatstroke

Let's start with heat cramps, which may progress to heat exhaustion, which may, in turn, progress to the most deadly form of heat-related illness: heatstroke.

Heat cramps are brief, often severe, muscle contractions that usually affect the legs, shoulders, and abdomen. Typically, heat cramps present in clusters as painful, hard lumps under the skin. They may occur during exercise, but, more typically, occur later when you're relaxing or taking a shower.

Heat cramps themselves are not serious, but the pain may be severe enough to require medical attention. More importantly, heat cramps may signal impending heat exhaustion, especially if they occur during strenuous, outdoor activity.

How do you treat heat cramps? Relax in a cool place and drink cold fluids, preferably one of the popular sports drinks. Do not take salt tablets. Salt tablets irritate the stomach and may induce nausea and vomiting, making the illness worse. Intravenous fluids are usually unnecessary unless the cramping is painful, frequent, and prolonged.

Our next stop on the gamut of heat-related illness is heat exhaustion. Heat exhaustion is caused by water depletion, salt depletion, or a combination of both. Water depletion occurs when a person is working, playing, or exercising in a hot environment and doesn't pause to drink adequate fluids. Children who rely on others for their fluid intake—especially children with medical problems such as mental retardation—are at risk for this type of heat exhaustion.

Salt depletion occurs when a person drinks plenty of water, but doesn't replace their salt loss. The signs and symptoms of heat exhaustion include the following:

- Headache
- Nausea
- Vomiting
- A mild fever

These signs and symptoms may also signal the onset of a viral illness, so it's important to distinguish between the two. Children with heat exhaustion may also complain of feeling weak or dizzy and act confused.

How do you treat heat exhaustion? As with heat cramps, move to a cool place and drink cold fluids. Milder cases can be treated with oral fluids and salty food if you aren't vomiting. But if there is any doubt about your condition, especially if the patient is a child, take her to the nearest emergency care facility for immediate treatment. She may require intravenous fluids and close monitoring for signs of impending heatstroke.

Now we come to heatstroke, the most serious, heat-related illness. It's an emergency condition.

Remember Korey Stringer, a lineman for the Minnesota Vikings? He suffered a fatal heatstroke during football practice in 2001. Remember, heatstroke can sneak up on you and kill.

Typically, you've already experienced some of the early signs and symptoms of heat exhaustion. But now, your temperature has jumped to 105 degrees or higher. You may feel confused and have dry skin, a rapid heart rate, and low blood pressure. Occasionally, patients have experienced a seizure as the first outward sign of heatstroke. If the cycle of rapid deterioration isn't broken, cardiovascular collapse ensues and death results.

The patient suffering from heatstroke needs emergency medical attention, including intravenous fluids and the application of rapid cooling techniques.

Remember, death from heatstroke is preventable. If you recognize the signs and symptoms of heat cramps and heat exhaustion early, and you treat them aggressively, you can prevent a fatal heatstroke.

A tip for the young athlete: Be aware of the warning signs of heat-related illness. If you, or a teammate, experience any of the following, stop what you're doing:

- Nausea
- Headache
- Dizziness
- Stumbling
- Any change in mental status, such as confusion

Find a cool place and drink cold fluids. Inform a parent or coach of your symptoms right away.

A final thought: Every summer, we read about a young child found dead after being left alone in a car on a hot day. The caregiver tells authorities, "I ran inside for just a minute." The temperature inside a car left parked in the sun—especially when the outside temperature is in the 80s or higher—can reach as high as 120 degrees within minutes and induce heatstroke in the occupant, particularly if he is a young child. Never, never leave a young child alone in a car, no matter what the season.

ARE 16-YEAR-OLDS MATURE ENOUGH TO DRIVE A CAR?

Talking to myself about deadly teen drivers:

    I: So what do you think?
  Me: About what?
    I: Today's question.
  Me: What question?
    I: Are 16-year-olds mature enough to drive a car?

Me: What brought this up?
I: Two lines of research, one based on fatality statistics, the other based on brain research.
Me: What do the statistics show?
I: Sixteen-year-olds are far worse drivers than older teens. For example, one in five 16-year-olds will have a reportable car crash within a year after passing their driver's test.
Me: Really?
I: Really. Also 16-year-old drivers are involved in fatal crashes at five times the rate of drivers 20 and older. In 2003, there were 937 16-year-old drivers involved in fatal crashes. In those crashes, 411 of the 16-year-old drivers died and 352 of their passengers were killed.
Me: I had no idea.
I: Studies also show that 16-year-olds make more driving errors, exceed speed limits, run off roads, and roll their vehicles at higher rates that any other age group. And their risk of dying nearly doubles when they drive at night or when you add a male passenger.
Me: Those are impressive statistics. How about the brain research?
I: Brain researchers at the National Institute of Health recently made an important discovery: The area of our brain that weighs risks, makes judgments, and controls impulsive behavior doesn't fully mature until we reach the age of 25.
Me: What's so important about that?
I: When a 16-year-old is driving 20 miles per hour over the speed limit, one part of her brain enjoys the thrill of going fast while the other part that's supposed to look over her shoulder and warn of negative consequences is useless. Researchers believe this reason explains why 16-year-old drivers crash at far higher rates than older drivers: They're

too immature to handle today's cars and highway risks, especially at night with friends in the car.
Me: I get it. So, where do we go from here?
I: In a recent Gallup poll, 61 percent of adults said they think a 16-year-old is too young to have a driver's license.
Me No kidding. That high?
I: Yep. And many states have begun restricting 16-year-old drivers by limiting how many passengers they can carry or banning late-night driving.
Me: So why not just raise the driving age to 17 or even 18?
I: That's easier said than done.
Me: How so?
I: Most students oppose raising the minimum driving age because they feel that responsible teen drivers shouldn't be punished for the mistakes of the small fraction who cause deadly crashes. Some parents oppose it too because they're tired of hauling their kids back and forth to school and other places.
Me: So convenience is more important than saving lives.

A further thought: This debate often stirs images of reckless teens driving drunk. But only about 10 percent of the 16-year-old drivers killed in 2003 had blood alcohol concentrations of 0.10 or higher, compared with 43 percent of 20- to 49-year-old drivers killed, according to the Insurance Institute for Highway Safety.

Ethical issues

SHOULD FAMILY MEMBERS BE ALLOWED IN THE ROOM DURING CPR?

Talking to myself after watching an episode of ER:

I: So what do you think?
Me: Think about what?
I: That awful scene.
Me: You mean the one where they were resuscitating the teenager with a gunshot wound, and his frantic mother walked in?
I: That's it. What did you think when Dr. Weaver pointed at her and yelled, "Get her out of here!"
Me: I didn't think much of it.
I: You didn't think much of it?
Me: Is there an echo in here?
I: It didn't bother you when they hustled the boy's mother out of the room?
Me: Not particularly.
I: It didn't bother you that the mother was not seen again until Dr. Weaver came out to tell her that her son was dead?
Me: But isn't that how it's always done?
I: Not always!
Me: You mean some doctors would let her stay in the room?
I: Yes.
Me: Name one.
I: Hey, I'm supposed to be asking the questions here.
Me: You're avoiding the issue; name one.
I: The doctors in the emergency room at Foote Hospital in Jackson, Michigan, have been doing it for 20 years.
Me: Really?
I: That's right. After family members in two separate incidents demanded to stay in the room, the hospital looked into it and decided to give it a try.
Me: How do they do it?
I: Family members are given the option of staying in the room. If they choose to stay, a chaplain or trained support person stays with them and helps them understand what's going on.

>   The staff has bought into it, and so has the community.
> **Me:** The hospital told the community?
> **I:** That's what I said.
> **Me:** Come to think about it, I guess it could be important, especially if the patient is likely to die.
> **I:** In one study, 83 percent of parents said they would want to be present during CPR if their child was likely to die.
> **Me:** Do the American Heart Association's guidelines for CPR mention this issue?
> **I:** The guidelines say, "Parents or family members seldom ask if they can be present unless they are encouraged to do so. Healthcare providers should offer the opportunity to family members whenever possible."
> **Me:** So a parent can hold her child's hand if she wants to?
> **I:** Yes, so a parent can hold her child's hand.

WOULD YOU TRY TO CONCEIVE A BABY TO SAVE A SIBLING'S LIFE?

Perhaps you remember back to 1991 when the Ayala family of Walnut, California, triggered a firestorm of criticism from ethicists and religious leaders after they revealed they had conceived a child, hopefully to be a stem cell donor for their 16-year-old daughter, Anissa, who was gradually dying of chronic myelogenous leukemia.

At the time, Anissa's brother, Airon, 18, and other relatives were not a match. So when Anissa's mother, Mary, had a dream in which she saw herself as the mother of three healthy children, she knew she had to have another baby. She believed it was the Lord telling her what to do.

But there was a problem: Mary's husband, Abraham, had undergone a vasectomy shortly after Anissa's birth; he could not father another child.

Mary finally convinced Abraham to try and have his vasectomy reversed, even though the odds of success were less than 10 percent. The reversal procedure worked, however, and Mary became pregnant the old-fashioned way, without using fertility drugs or in vitro fertilization. Still another problem remained, however: The chance that a new brother or sister would be a stem cell match was only 25 percent.

After Anissa's new sister, Marissa-Eve, was born, doctors found she was a perfect match. Today, 31-year-old Anissa Alaya is fully recovered and working as assistant director of the Bone Marrow Donor Program for the American Red Cross, Southern California region. Her sister is a happy, healthy 13-year-old with no memory of the stem cell donation she gave, saving her older sister's life. And Mary and Abraham Alaya are the proud parents of three healthy children, a dream come true.

More recently, medical scientists in Chicago have taken the "Alaya method" several steps further, using the latest reproductive techniques to create healthy babies for use as stem-cell donors for their ailing brothers and sisters.

In a recent issue of the *Journal of the American Medical Association*, doctors at the Reproductive Genetics Institute in Chicago reported the births of five perfectly matched children, who had been conceived in order to use the stem cells from their cord blood to save a sibling's life. Their siblings suffered from several types of leukemia and a rare form of anemia, known as Diamond-Blackfan anemia, which is often fatal.

For the first time, in vitro fertilization, combined with preimplantation genetic diagnosis and embryo tissue-typing, had all been used before inserting the embryo in the uterus and establishing a pregnancy.

Walking the Baby Beat

By now, most of us know about in vitro fertilization. But just in case, here's a simplified version of how it works:

- You place an egg and some sperm together in a petri dish.
- Then you wait for fertilization to take place and for the resulting single cell to begin multiplying over several days.
- Once you have a four- to eight-cell embryo, you place it in the uterus and hope for implantation and a successful pregnancy.

Preimplantation genetic diagnosis is a method of testing the embryo for genetic disease while embryo tissue-typing allows you to compare the embryo's tissue type to a diseased child's tissue type and see whether they match. Here's how they work:

- You pluck a single cell from the four- to eight-cell embryo and test it for a variety of genetic diseases, such as Down syndrome.
- If the single cell passes that test, you then perform embryo tissue-typing on the cell and compare those results to the tissue type of the embryo's afflicted sibling to see whether the two types match.
- If they match, you insert the embryo (minus the tested cell) in the uterus and let nature takes its course.
- Hopefully, the mother will give birth nine months later to a baby whose custom-made stem cells contained in its cord blood can be transfused intravenously (transplanted) into the afflicted sibling and cure the disease.

This growing practice of creating healthy babies so they can serve as stem cell donors for their ailing brothers and sisters is highly controversial. Some ethicists and religious leaders have labeled the practice "a search-and-destroy mission," and "morally troubling."

Why? Because those embryos found to have a genetic disease and those embryos that don't match, are usually discarded.

What would you do if your 16-year-old daughter had leukemia, and her only hope was a stem cell transplant, and a suitable donor wasn't available? Would you use this procedure to try to conceive a baby to serve as a stem cell donor for your afflicted child, hoping to save her life?

ARE WE DOING THE RIGHT THING?

Q *Six months ago, after my wife found out she was pregnant, a prenatal test showed the baby had cystic fibrosis. Now, my wife's sister and brother-in-law are planning to start a family and might also be at risk. We haven't shared the test results with them because if anyone knew we carry the gene for cystic fibrosis, our job prospects and health insurance might be jeopardized. Are we doing the right thing or just being selfish?*

A The brave new world of genetic technology is full of choices no one has ever had to make before. In this case, you and your wife have a right to privacy. But you also have a moral obligation to pass along the test results to your wife's sister and brother-in-law so they can consider that information when making their reproductive choices. If the tables were turned and your wife's sister and brother-in-law were in your shoes, what would you want them to do?

In my opinion, your moral obligation to help your wife's sister and brother-in-law outweighs your right to privacy, despite the slight insurance and employment risks. Besides, won't they eventually find out that your child has cystic fibrosis? What will you say when the discussion turns to how you found out about the diagnosis? Will you tell them the truth or will you make up a lie to save face?

SHOULD THE MEDICAL TEAM HAVE TRIED TO SEPARATE THESE CONJOINED TWINS?

Talking to myself about the Bijani twins, who were 29 years old and joined at the head:

I: So what do you think about the failed attempt to separate Laleh and Ladan now?
Me: I'm not sure.
I: I thought you had an opinion about everything.
Me: Stuff it, wise guy!
I: Sorry. I shouldn't have said that.
Me: I'm sorry too. It's just that I'm still upset by their deaths.
I: May I try again?
Me: Okay.
I: Knowing the operation carried huge risks, did the medical team do the right thing by trying to separate Laleh and Ladan Bijani?
Me: I think so.
I: Why?
Me: Laleh and Ladan were aware of the operation's risks, right?
I: Right.
Me: Yet they pressed for the surgery anyway.
I: I know, but why?
Me: Because they desperately wanted something we take for granted—living as single human beings.
I: Are you saying those doctors were simply order-takers, like a waitress in a restaurant?
Me: Of course not! This case was special. None of us can fully understand what it's like to live for 29 years, joined at the head by an identical twin.

They wanted to finally sleep in their own beds, to walk side by side, to live out their dreams, to have separate careers, to marry and have children.
I: Go on.
Me: I believe that Laleh and Ladan were saying enough is enough; we can't go on like this. Though we love each other very much, we cherish our freedom to live out our hopes and dreams even more.
I: Even if the risky surgery failed, costing them their lives?
Me: Yes.
I: One of the doctors now says the operation to separate Laleh and Ladan should have been done in stages.
Me: I know. And if there is a next time, the operation may be done that way.
I: So even though the operation failed, a lot was learned to perhaps help others?
Me: That's right. Medical progress is measured not only by ups, but also by downs, and sometimes even death.
I: So you think those two young women sincerely believed they were doing the right thing, whether they lived or died?
Me: I do. I also believe they wouldn't want those doctors spending the rest of their lives feeling guilty and remorseful. They would want them, instead, to move on, using what they've learned to help others.
I: A noble thought.
Me: From two noble sisters.

WHEN A CURE FOR MOTHER'S CANCER THREATENS HER UNBORN BABY

Imagine this scenario: You're 38 years old and finally pregnant for the first time after undergoing two years of fertility treatments. Then three weeks after learning the good news, you and your husband sit in a surgeon's office as he tells you the lump you found in your breast is malignant. You're given a one in four chance of surviving five years.

You leave the office still tearless. But that night you break down and sob away in your husband's arms.

Your case is reviewed by two highly respected panels of cancer specialists who advise treatment for difficult cancer cases. Both panels recommend the same plan:

- Therapeutic abortion
- Mastectomy
- Chemotherapy
- Radiation
- Tamoxifen hormonal therapy

Both groups of doctors are concerned, primarily, with saving your life. With your pregnancy out of the way, the rising hormonal levels of pregnancy, which could encourage cancer growth, would not be a factor. Treatment could be more aggressive and started sooner. They believe this approach offers you the best chance for survival.

Your own obstetrician and oncologist, however, take a different tack: They found several case reports of pregnant women who delivered healthy babies after delaying chemotherapy until after 14 weeks, when fetal organs and limbs had formed. They believe this approach offers a reasonable risk for the baby and an effective treatment for you.

Which path should you choose? Can you give up this pregnancy? Are you prepared to give your life for your child's? Are you willing to raise a child with birth defects? Is your husband willing to be a single parent? These and many other questions fill your late-night discussions and finally force you to make a rule: no cancer talk after 8 P.M.

Your surgeon removes your left breast three weeks after the first biopsy results. Confirming the aggressiveness of the cancer, 5 of the 13 axillary lymph nodes are invaded by cancer cells. Still, you decide to fight your cancer while trying to save your baby.

At 14 weeks of your pregnancy, you begin six months of chemotherapy, delivered at three week intervals. The plan is to finish the treatments a few weeks before the baby is due. Radiation will begin after you deliver your baby.

You grapple with overwhelming exhaustion from the chemo every third week. But your baby is growing normally, and, despite your oncologist's prediction, you don't loose your hair.

Finally, you give birth four weeks early, after a five-hour labor and natural delivery. You cuddle your long-awaited son, Tanner, to your remaining breast. Seven days later, you undergo the last chemo treatment then move on to radiation.

This was the situation faced, and path taken, by Jana Striegel-Wilson back in 1994. Writing her own story in *The New York Times,* Streigel-Wilson continued her battle with cancer.

Two years after giving birth to Tanner, the cancer returned. Despite another round of aggressive treatment, a biopsy showed that the cancer remained in her sternum and was growing. So surgeons at the M.D. Anderson Cancer Center in Houston removed her sternum and replaced it with a new strong-as-bone plastic one. Now, after a painful recovery, she is writing children's books and enjoying her 11-year-old son. "Tanner is articulate, delightfully curious and kicks a mean soccer ball," says his mother.

Would terminating her pregnancy have prevented the recurrence and improved her chances of survival? "The medical community has mixed opinions," says Striegel-Wilson. "But regardless of my final outcome, I know I would not have done anything differently."

SHOULD THE FEDERAL GOVERNMENT FUND EMBRYONIC STEM CELL RESEARCH?

Talking to myself about the frustrating debate over funding for embryonic stem cell research:

I: It's disgusting!
Me: What's disgusting?
I: The current debate over whether the federal government should spend taxpayers' money to support embryonic stem cell research.
Me: But didn't the House of Representatives recently vote to allow federal funding for research on stem cells taken from unused embryos at fertility clinics?
I: As a matter of fact, it was just last week.
Me: And isn't it possible that stem cells from those unused embryos might one day be used to repair organs or tissues impaired by illnesses such as diabetes, spinal cord injury, or degenerative diseases such as Parkinson's and Alzheimer's ?
I: That's correct.
Me: In fact, haven't some cases of Parkinson's disease been successfully treated by implanting fetal cells into the patient's brain?
I: Right you are, old swami.
Me: And don't couples undergoing these fertility procedures normally create more embryos than they plan to use in trying to produce a child?
I: Almost always. That's why fertility specialists estimate 150,000 or more frozen embryos are currently stored in the United States alone.
Me: And most of them will eventually be discarded?
I: Right again, my alter ego.

Me: So now the House has proposed a solution. What's so disgusting about that?
I: You forgot one small item.
Me: What's that?
I: President Bush vowed to veto the bill passed by the House.
Me: Even though most of the frozen embryos will be destroyed anyway?
I: Right again, knucklehead.
Me: Are you sure? Did he actually say that?
I: Here's the quote: "I made it very clear to Congress that the use of federal money, taxpayers' money, to promote science which destroys life in order to save life is—I'm against that."
Me: What about research using adult stem cells and stem cells from umbilical cord blood?
I: The House also approved a less controversial bill encouraging research using stem cells from those two sources.
Me: So all isn't lost.
I: Some private funding sources are also stepping up and attempting to fill the void left by the federal government on human embryonic stem cells.
Me: So, like I said, things are not as bad as they might seem.
I: Except for another small item.
Me: What now?
I: There's a difference between embryonic stem cells and stem cells from cord blood or adults. Embryonic stem cells are totipotent, meaning they have the potential to become almost any organ or tissue. On the other hand, cord blood stem cells and adult stem cells, especially, have a more limited potential for healing and repair.
Me: But so many of the frozen embryos are going to be discarded anyway.
I: Sad, isn't it?
Me: Especially if a loved one is crippled by one of those awful diseases you mentioned and can't get help.

WHEN A CHILD WITH DOWN SYNDROME OUTLIVES HIS PARENTS

Q *My sister and her husband are both in their early 40s. They have one child. He's three years old and was born with Down syndrome. Other than the usual colds and ear infections that children get, he seems pretty healthy. I'm 38, and my husband and I have two girls who are nine and six. Can you tell me how long the typical child with Down syndrome is expected to live? I ask because my greatest fear is that my nephew will outlive both his parents and my husband and I, possibly leaving his care later on to one or both of our daughters.*

A Due to advances in the surgical correction of heart defects and in the treatment of common infections, the average life expectancy of a person affected by Down syndrome now exceeds 60 years. This relatively long life expectancy has meant that younger family members are almost invariably left with the burden of caring for a family member with Down syndrome. If no one is willing to do it, the state usually takes on that responsibility.

If you haven't already done so, you and your sister might consider sitting down with your husbands to draw up a tentative plan for your nephew's care should something unforeseen happen to his parents. Then the four of you can revisit your tentative plan, from time to time, as the years go by.

A further thought: How a couple reacts to the birth of a baby with Down syndrome as well as how they react to the important issue you raised here will vary from couple to couple. Don't assume anything!

For instance, your sister and her husband may be in synch with each other. They may both dearly love your nephew and be equally involved in raising him. So far, so good.

But when it comes to discussing his long-term future, their views may differ widely. One parent may not want to talk about it while the other may disagree. And even if they happen to both agree that it's a good idea to plan ahead, people often change their minds later on as circumstances change. This possibility reinforces the value of getting together, from time to time, to reevaluate your tentative plan.

Now, let's suppose everything goes smoothly for the next 15 years. You and your sister are still married to the same men, the four of you are still in good health, your daughters are now 24 and 21 years old, and your nephew has remained healthy too. Is it right to expect your daughters to feel a responsibility toward their cousin's care if the need should arise? Is it right to even ask them to participate, if needed? What if they express doubts? What if they don't want to get involved?

How will you and your husband, as well as your sister and her husband, react to those kinds of responses? Some families have handled this kind of situation without tearing the families apart. Others have not been so fortunate. Wending your way through the maze of possibilities, over the years, will require thoughtful and considerate understanding from all involved, not an easy task.

Most people aren't ready to talk about these issues during the first few years after a child with Down syndrome is born. But, sooner or later, they must be faced. Good for you for bringing it up now.

BABY'S RESUSCITATION RAISES TROUBLING ETHICAL ISSUES

The following story is true.

Conor Shamus McInnerney was born at Olympic Memorial Hospital in Port Angeles, Washington, in January 1998. He was discharged from the hospital two days later. On the third day of life, in the early evening, while feeding at his mother's breast, Conor suddenly stopped breathing, turned blue and did not respond to stimulation.

The paramedics were called and arrived minutes later. They also found that Conor was unresponsive. He had no spontaneous respirations, no heartbeat, and no recordable blood pressure. His pupils were fixed and dilated.

The paramedics inserted a breathing tube down Conor's throat and started CPR. They then transported Conor by ambulance through a blinding snowstorm to the hospital where he was born.

Upon arriving at the hospital emergency room, Conor's condition was unchanged and CPR was continued. Treatment included chest compressions, assisted ventilation, resuscitative drugs, and intravenous fluids.

Approximately 40 minutes after starting CPR, a pulse was recorded for the first time. Minutes later, Conor's pediatrician, Dr. Eugene Turner, arrived and assumed responsibility for the baby's care.

CPR was continued for another 50 minutes. Dr. Turner then discussed Conor's poor prognosis with his parents, and, together, they decided to stop resuscitative measures. The parents held their lifeless baby for a short time, then he was pronounced dead.

Conor's parents had already left for home when an emergency-room nurse, who happened by the room, noticed that the baby was making infrequent gasping efforts. Touching Conor's chest, she thought she felt a heartbeat. But when Dr. Turner rechecked the baby, his pupils were still fixed and dilated.

Dr. Turner stimulated the baby by rubbing his back, but Conor's only response was to continue the gasping movements. Dr. Turner said he thought the baby would stop gasping soon. So he left the hospital and headed out in the snowstorm, on foot, for home.

A short time later, Dr. Turner was called at home and told that an emergency-room physician was working on the baby. His heart rate had picked up, and his color was pinker. Dr. Turner asked the caller not to notify the baby's parents; he would come back in.

Upon his return, Dr. Turner continued working on the baby. By now, it was almost midnight. More than four hours had passed since Conor first turned blue and stopped breathing at home. Finally, Dr. Turner concluded that Conor was brain dead and covered his mouth and nose with a hand. The gasping stopped, and Conor was pronounced dead again.

Two nurses, who were in the room at the time of Conor's death, couldn't believe their eyes. To them, Dr. Turner's action was unbelievable. But what should they do?

Rumors that Dr. Turner, the town's most beloved pediatrician, had smothered a baby spread through the hospital like wildfire. Olympic Memorial's executive committee met three days later and decided to ask the state Medical Quality Assurance Commission to investigate. The Commission met in emergency session and decided to restrict Dr. Turner's license, ordering him not to make any decisions to stop patient resuscitation. The county prosecutor then got involved.

Folks in the town of 19,000 were deeply divided in their views about Dr. Turner's treatment of Conor. Some felt strongly that Dr. Turner had killed the baby by blocking his air passages. They wanted Dr. Turner charged with murder.

Others felt just as deeply that Dr. Turner had done the compassionate thing, not wanting the baby to suffer any longer. Still others were not so sure. Dr. Turner had tried hard, perhaps too hard, to save the baby. But his blocking the baby's airway disturbed them.

On September 1, 1998, almost nine months after Conor McInnerney's death, the county prosecutor concluded that the baby was not brain dead when Dr. Turner placed his hand over the baby's nose and mouth, causing the baby's death. The prosecutor then charged Dr. Turner with second-degree murder.

Three months later, a special prosecutor was appointed to take over the case. But two months later, in a dramatic turn of events, the charges against Dr. Turner were dropped. The special prosecutor didn't think he could prove the second-degree murder charge, which requires showing intent.

This disturbing case raises several questions:

- **Were the efforts to resuscitate Conor excessive?**

Experienced observers would say the efforts to resuscitate Conor, which lasted several hours, were excessive. Fortunately, we now have nationally recognized guidelines that address this issue for newborns. If a baby's heart beat is still absent after a complete resuscitation has lasted for 10 minutes, those efforts may be stopped.

- **Did Conor receive appropriate treatment?**

This question is slightly different from the first one. Up until he was pronounced dead the first time, Conor apparently received appropriate, though excessive, treatment. But the treatment he received after that was clearly inappropriate. When a baby is pronounced dead, especially after undergoing prolonged resuscitative efforts, his doctor should advise parents and staff that occasionally such babies may subsequently experience episodes of gasping or have a detectable heart beat. These are terminal events, part of the dying process, not an indication to resume CPR. Even though it may be difficult emotionally for those standing nearby, it's a mistake to resume resuscitative efforts when events like this occur. Someone should wrap the baby in a blanket and hold him until the gasping and heart beat stops.

- **Was Conor brain dead when Dr. Turner placed his hand over the baby's mouth and nose to stop the baby's gasping?**

Brain death is defined as the irreversible loss of whole brain function. Some brain stem function is required for a patient to make gasping movements, therefore Dr. Turner was incorrect. Conor was not brain dead. Was he irreversibly brain-damaged? Yes.

- **Was it appropriate for Dr. Turner to place his hand over Conor's nose and mouth to stop his gasping?**

No. It is inappropriate to hasten the dying process of anyone by occluding the airway. Again, all of this could have been avoided had Dr. Turner simply wrapped Conor in a blanket, took Conor in his arms, sat down in a chair, and held him until Conor's gasping and fluttering heart had stopped.

Easy for me to say now, in retrospect?
Certainly easier than it must have been for Dr. Turner and all concerned back then.

Bonus Section

MY HEROES

It gives me great pleasure to introduce you to eight outstanding people, five of them medical pioneers, in this special collection of articles called "My Heroes." Each of them spoke to me inwardly, sharing the same conflicts, passions, and hopes and dreams. That's when I made a startling discovery: I had more in common with them than I ever thought possible. Their journeys were much like my own journey. Aha!

This simple discovery, repeated many times, changed my life. Perhaps you'll be this lucky too.

Contents

- The newborn APGAR score: Just one of Dr. Virginia Apgar's many achievements
- Dr. Albert Schweitzer: The renowned humanitarian who showed me the way
- The hidden talent of Dr. Spock
- Frieda Pushnik: "The armless and legless wonder"
- Franklin Delano Roosevelt: Rescued at birth
- Dr. Ignaz Semmelweis: "You must wash your hands!"
- Dr. Martin A. Couney: "The incubator-baby doctor"
- Suddenly paraplegic, Joseph Stock never gave up

D. Gary Benfield, M.D.

THE NEWBORN APGAR SCORE: JUST ONE OF DR. VIRGINIA APGAR'S MANY ACHIEVEMENTS

"Every baby born in a hospital, anywhere in the world, is first seen through the eyes of Virginia Apgar."
—An anonymous physician

It had been a long and difficult labor, even as first-time births go. Then one last push, and Cindy Martin's little girl was born.

I was examining the baby in the delivery room when her mother suddenly sat up on one elbow.

"What were my baby's APGAR scores?" she whispered anxiously.

"Her one-minute score was 9, and her five-minute score was 10," I said. "She lost one point for color. Your daughter's doing fine."

She thanked me and dropped off to sleep, still smiling.

Thanks to childbirth education classes and a steady stream of baby care books, most parents know about the APGAR score. In fact, some parents like Cindy ask for their baby's scores before asking how much their baby weighs. But even though most of us know about the score, few know much about the pioneering doctor who invented it.

Virginia Apgar was born in Westfield, New Jersey, in 1909, the year after Henry Ford introduced the Model T. A curious, energetic, and fast-talking child, she learned to read at the age of three and started taking violin lessons when she was six.

At Westfield High, Virginia played violin in the orchestra, ran for the track team, played basketball and tennis, and competed on the debate team. She also taught herself to speak Greek and loved collecting stamps. "How does she do it?" asked the Westfield High yearbook. "The duty of the bee is second only to that of Virginia."

Walking the Baby Beat

Only 16, she entered Mount Holyoke College, determined to become a doctor. But her biggest problem was finding the time to fit everything in. She played on 11 class teams and seven varsity teams, wrote for the newspaper, acted, played violin in the orchestra, opened the college library every morning, took care of the anatomy lab, and earned extra money during Christmas vacations selling linens and catching cats for the zoology department. Along the way, she got accepted to the College of Physicians and Surgeons at Columbia University.

Virginia started medical school one month before the 1929 stock market crash. Four years later, she graduated fourth in her class and nearly $4,000 in debt, an enormous sum for a self-supporting woman facing more years of training in an internship that would pay almost nothing.

With her sights set on becoming a surgeon, she won a highly competitive, two-year surgical internship at Columbia Presbyterian Hospital. But midway through her training, her department chairman, Dr. Allen Whipple, suggested she switch her career plans from surgery to anesthesiology.

After a great deal of soul-searching, Dr. Apgar reluctantly decided to take Dr. Whipple's advice. But first, she insisted on completing her surgical internship, making her a fully trained surgeon.

After two years of additional training in anesthesiology, Dr. Apgar, 29, was appointed by Dr. Whipple to head up the division of anesthesiology, under the department of surgery, at Columbia Presbyterian Hospital. She was the first woman physician to head up a division of any kind in the medical school's history.

Under Dr. Apgar's guidance, the division of anesthesiology gained a reputation as one of the best in the nation:

- Medical students were taught anesthesia for the first time.
- An anesthesia residency training program was started.

- Nurse anesthetists were gradually replaced in the operating room with physician anesthesiologists.
- At one point, Dr. Apgar directed the work of 33 residents and 10 anesthesiologists.

During World War II, Dr. Apgar and her short-handed staff worked extra long hours just to keep up with the clinical load, leaving no time for research. She had no idea that her lack of published research would soon come back to haunt her.

After the war was over, in 1949, Dr. Apgar's division of anesthesiology was split off from the surgery department and became a separate department. However, she was unexpectedly passed over for chair of the new department.

Wanting to recruit someone with a strong background in research, the search committee chose Dr. E. M. Papper from Bellevue to head up the new department. Dr. Apgar was promoted to full professor, however, making her the first woman full professor in the medical school's history.

Forever the optimist, Dr. Apgar charged ahead, turning her energy and skills to the labor and delivery area and obstetrical anesthesia.

One morning, later in 1949, the anesthesia staff was gathered in the hospital cafeteria for breakfast when a curious medical student asked Dr. Apgar a question about the best way to evaluate newborns immediately after birth.

Dr. Apgar was well aware that physicians only had two ways to evaluate a baby's condition at birth: the time from birth to the first cry and the time from birth to the first breath. She also knew that neither approach accurately reflected a baby's true condition. As a result, it was difficult to tell when a baby needed help, and it was difficult to study the effects of childbirth anesthesia on the baby and get reliable results.

In response to the medical student's question, Dr. Apgar reached for the nearest piece of paper and jotted down the five vital signs she often used to monitor patients while they were under anesthesia:

- Heart rate
- Breathing effort
- Reflexes
- Muscle tone
- Color

She then scooped up the list and headed for the delivery area, eager to see whether she could use the items on her list to help evaluate babies shortly after birth.

Still carrying a full clinical load, Dr. Apgar spent the next two years attending hundreds of deliveries, observing and recording each baby's vital signs. Then she devised a method of "scoring" each baby's condition by assigning zero, one, or two points to each of the five signs. In effect, a baby's score could range from 0 to 10. After much trial and error, she decided to score each baby at one minute after birth.

Her new scoring system was published in a highly respected medical journal in 1953, the same year James Watson and Francis Crick proposed the double helix structure for DNA. And before long, hospitals throughout the country—and eventually all over the world—began using her scoring system routinely.

"I remember one of our nurse anesthetists bringing Dr. Apgar's article in and we liked it," said Murdina Desmond, M.D., former professor of pediatrics at Baylor University in Houston, and now deceased. "All we had before that was the crying time and the breathing time to tell us how a baby was doing at birth. They were terrible indicators! We started using her scoring system right away at Jefferson Davis Hospital in Houston.

"A short time later, Virginia visited us in Houston," continued Dr. Desmond. "I showed her a poster drawn up by one of our medical students before her system was published. In the center it showed a newborn in the delivery room. In the upper right hand corner the baby's pediatrician was sitting in his office at a desk. In the upper left hand corner the mother's obstetrician was leaving the hospital. There was no doctor for the baby. The caption read, 'I'm Nobody's Baby.' Dr. Apgar chuckled, obviously pleased at what she had accomplished."

Now everything changed, for the newborn and for Dr. Apgar.

- The newborn was no longer "Nobody's Baby." Physicians now regarded each baby as a patient with its own assigned examiner.
- Now Dr. Apgar had the tool she needed to study the effects of obstetrical anesthesia on newborn babies.

Armed with her newborn scoring system, she launched a series of studies that transformed obstetrical anesthesia into a specialty all its own.

One study involved cyclopropane, Dr. Apgar's favorite anesthetic. After comparing the one- and five-minute scores for babies born under regional anesthesia to those born under cyclopropane, she was shocked to discover that babies born under cyclopropane were much more depressed. So the next day she announced, "There goes my favorite gas." As a result, cyclopropane rapidly fell out of favor for use in childbirth.

"Modern obstetrical anesthesia was born, all because of Ginny," said S. H. Ngai, M.D., professor emeritus in anesthesiology at Columbia. "Columbia Presbyterian became the mecca of obstetrical anesthesia. During the 1950s, almost all of the nation's prominent obstetric anesthesiologists were Ginny's students."

During the course of her career, Dr. Apgar trained an estimated 250 anesthesiologists. She herself administered the anesthetic for more than 20,000 operations and the delivery of some 17,000 babies.

But medicine was only part of Virginia Apgar's life. An enthusiastic stamp collector, she gathered stamps from all over the world, bringing them home for her stamp-collecting friends.

She loved music, fishing, gardening, and baseball (the Brooklyn Dodgers was her team), drove a fire-engine red convertible and, later in life, learned to fly. She was an accomplished cellist and violist, and built her own stringed instruments. She often carried her handmade viola to medical conferences around the world, playing chamber music with old friends and new acquaintances.

"My first glimpse of Virginia Apgar was in 1956 when she dashed into my room for a pre-op visit," recalled Carleen Hutchins, noted maker of stringed instruments and an authority on the acoustics of stringed instruments. "My surgeon had suggested I bring along one of the violas I had made to show to my anesthesiologist. After the checkup, Virginia played the viola in my room, much to the delight of the whole floor!"

Mrs. Hutchins and Dr. Apgar began talking about making violas—by then one of Dr. Apgar's many interests. Mrs. Hutchins told her she had seen a maple shelf in a telephone booth down the hall that seemed well-seasoned and ideal for making a viola.

While Mrs. Hutchins convalesced, she and Dr. Apgar made plans to remove the shelf and replace it with a copy made of plywood.

Dr. Apgar bought the plywood replacement and brought it to the hospital. A friend supplied a crowbar and a saw. Then late one night, as Mrs. Hutchins' husband stood guard, the two women pried away the maple shelf and replaced it with the plywood board. Dr. Apgar kept the original and, with the help of Mrs. Hutchins, turned it into the back of the viola she carried with her to medical meetings around the world.

D. Gary Benfield, M.D.

For the next 18 years, until Dr. Apgar's death, the two women remained the best of friends.

In 1959, at the age of 50, Dr. Apgar used a sabbatical leave from Columbia to earn a master's degree in public health at Johns Hopkins University. But instead of returning to Columbia as originally planned, she launched a new career as medical director of the newly formed Birth Defects Section of the March of Dimes. Under her leadership, the March of Dimes successfully shifted its mission from eliminating polio to preventing and treating birth defects.

Meanwhile, in 1962, two Denver pediatricians, Drs. Butterfield and Covey, paid tribute to Dr. Apgar's newborn scoring system in a short article they wrote for the *Journal of the American Medical Association.* In an effort to make her scoring system easier to remember, the authors identified the five variables of her scoring system (color, heart rate, reflex irritability, muscle tone, and respiratory effort) with the five letters of her last name. (A for appearance, P for pulse, G for grimace, A for activity, and R for respiration.). As a result, her newborn scoring system became known as the APGAR score, and it was easier to remember.

In her job with the March of Dimes, Dr. Apgar traveled the world, working closely with dozens of leading scientists who were investigating the causes and treatments of birth defects. During those trips, she always found time to meet with parent and professional groups. But what she discovered in those meetings disturbed her: Parents had lots of questions about birth defects, but physicians avoided answering them. In effect, the subject of birth defects was locked away in the closet.

Determined to unlock the closet and bring the subject out in the open, Dr. Apgar teamed up with Joan Beck, noted columnist for the *Chicago Tribune,* and wrote the book, *Is My Baby All Right?: A 1973 Guide to Birth Defects.*

With her new book under her arm, she carried her message all over the world, speaking to medical groups, parent groups, and to anyone else who would listen. Her revolutionary book helped remove the stigma attached to children with birth defects, changing the way society viewed these children and their parents. "Dr. Apgar always saw the child within," said Dr. Joseph Butterfield. "To her the birth defect was secondary."

Virginia Apgar received numerous awards during her lifetime:

- The Alumni Association of the College of Physicians and Surgeons at Columbia University awarded her its gold medal for distinguished service in medicine—the first woman ever to receive the honor.
- The *Ladies Home Journal* included her among the first eight winners of its "Women of the Year" awards.
- The American Society of Anesthesiology awarded her its distinguished service award.
- She received the New York Infirmary's Elizabeth Blackwell citation for distinguished service to medicine by a woman.
- She also received honorary degrees from the Women's Medical College of Pennsylvania; Mount Holyoke College; The New Jersey School of Medicine and Dentistry; Boston University; and Russell Sage College.

Dr. Apgar worked for the March of Dimes right up to the end of her life. She died of cancer on August 7, 1974, at Columbia Presbyterian Hospital, where she had trained and worked for 30 years. A memorial service attended by thousands of colleagues and admirers was held five weeks later at Riverside Church in New York City.

Ten years later, Dr. Joseph Butterfield, one of the two Denver pediatricians who proposed naming Dr. Apgar's newborn scoring system the APGAR score and whose daughter was born with spina bifida, sparked a movement to honor Virginia Apgar with a U.S. postage stamp. More than a dozen national organizations, including the American Academy of Pediatrics and the March of Dimes, joined together in the campaign.

The 20-cent Virginia Apgar stamp was issued in Dallas, Texas on October 24, 1994, at the annual meeting of the American Academy of Pediatrics.

In a ceremony described as "a love fest," the Apgar String Quartet played music on instruments built by Virginia Apgar. The four stringed instruments were later acquired by Columbia University College of Physicians and Surgeons where they are currently maintained and displayed.

More than 30 years have passed since Virginia Apgar's death, yet her influence lives on. Like Cindy Martin's newborn daughter, every baby born in a hospital, anywhere in the world, is first seen through the eyes of Virginia Apgar.

Acknowledgment

A number of sources were used for this article, including the following:

- Personal interviews with Joan Beck, Murdina Desmond, M.D., and Joseph Butterfield, M.D.
- Joan Beck, "Virginia Apgar, in memoriam" in *Clinical Perinatology,* 2nd ed., Silvio Aladjem, Audrey Brown, and Claude Sureau (eds.) (St. Louis: The C.V. Mosby Company, 1980), pp. xix–xxix.
- The writings of Dr. Selma Calmes, anesthesiologist and medical historian.

DR. ALBERT SCHWEITZER: THE RENOWNED HUMANITARIAN WHO SHOWED ME THE WAY

Before I introduce Dr. Schweitzer, let me tell you a bit about myself and how we met. Then you'll understand how he became one of my favorite heroes.

Walking the Baby Beat

I was born in Concord, North Carolina, shortly before World War II. But I grew up in a housing project in Baltimore, Maryland.

I attended Baltimore Polytechnic Institute, an all-boys, public high school, where I received an education second to none.

We took classes in trigonometry, algebra, geometry, calculus, physics, chemistry, English, American history, a foreign language, technical drawing, surveying, woodworking, pattern making, and metal work. We were also taught how to use the slide rule; we didn't have calculators or computers back then.

Our unofficial dress code? "Every good Poly boy wears a tie." I also played tuba in the marching band.

How far back was this? The early 1950s, when Dwight Eisenhower was president and Richard Nixon was vice president.

After graduating from Poly, I majored in electrical engineering at the University of Maryland in College Park, where I once again played tuba in the marching band.

During my freshman year, Maryland played Oklahoma in the Orange Bowl. Traveling to Miami by train, the band marched in the Orange Bowl parade the night before the big game, and performed at halftime. The theme of our halftime show was "Rock Around the Clock." You know, "One o'clock, two o'clock, three o'clock, rock" and so on. Maryland lost the game, but we had such a good time it really didn't matter.

After graduating from Maryland in 1959, I went to work for an engineering firm in Georgetown, D.C., just a few blocks from John and Jackie Kennedy's townhouse. But it didn't take more than a few months for me to realize electrical engineering wasn't for me. I wanted a career that involved directly helping people. So I started thinking about the possibilities.

I thought seriously enough about teaching math or science to junior or senior high school students that I interviewed with several school districts. But even though I had more math credits under my belt than anyone teaching math in their schools, they all required a degree in education. I offered to take education courses at night while teaching during the day, but they still turned me down.

One afternoon, I was window shopping in downtown Baltimore when a book on display in a Cokesbury Bookstore window caught my eye and pulled me inside.

A wrinkled, older man, who had a full head of white hair, a bushy white mustache, and sad, but thoughtful, eyes, looked out at me from the book's cover. I couldn't resist that face, so I bought the book, *Out of My Life and Thought,* which was written by the man on the cover, Albert Schweitzer. I had no way of knowing he and his book were about to change my life.

Albert Schweitzer was born on January 14, 1875, in Kayserberg, Germany, now a part of France. His father and maternal grandfather were both ministers, and both grandfathers played the organ.

As a youngster, Albert studied the piano and the organ, even before his legs were long enough to reach the pedals. He was only nine when he first substituted for the regular organist at his father's church in Gunsbach.

As a young man, and until his middle eighties, he had a distinguished musical career, playing the organ in concert all over the world. He also wrote a biography in French about Johann Sebastian Bach; published a book on organ building and organ playing; and rewrote the Bach book in German.

When he was 18, he entered the University of Strasbourg where he studied theology, philosophy, and musical theory. A year later, he interrupted his studies to fulfill a one-year commitment to serve in the German infantry.

At the age of 21, Schweitzer decided what he was going to do with the rest of his life:

- He would study science, music, and theology for nine more years.
- Then he would devote the rest of his life to directly serving humanity.

Walking the Baby Beat

In 1899, when he was 24, Schweitzer earned a Ph.D. in philosophy from the University of Strasbourg. That same year, he also published a book based on his Ph.D. thesis: *Kant's Philosophy of Religion*. The following year he earned a degree in theology and found time to publish a second book, *The Mystery of the Kingdom of God*. Soon after that, he was appointed to the permanent faculty of the local theological seminary.

When he turned 30, Schweitzer kept the promise he had made to himself and decided to become a doctor, devoting the rest of his life to treating the natives of South Africa. He resigned from the seminary and was admitted in 1906 to the University of Strasbourg School of Medicine.

During his freshman year of medical school, Schweitzer published his biography of Bach in French. The following year, he published one of his best-known books, *The Quest of the Historical Jesus,* and a second book on organ building and organ playing. He frequently pushed himself to the point of exhaustion while juggling his medical studies and writing his books.

During his internship, Schweitzer married Helene Bresslau, daughter of a well-known Strasbourg historian. Six months later, he finished his internship and was awarded the degree of doctor of medicine.

On March 26, 1913, Dr. Albert Schweitzer and his wife sailed for Africa, where, aided by the Paris Missionary Society, he started a hospital in Lambarene. Although he would travel back and forth to Europe and to other parts of the world more than a dozen times during the rest of his life, he always returned to Lambarene and the African people who sought his help there.

During those years, Albert Schweitzer the doctor, musician, philosopher, theologian, humanitarian, author, and spokesperson for world peace rang up a long list of accomplishments and awards. A few of them are listed here:

- Schweitzer preached reverence for life, the guiding principle behind his *Philosophy of Civilization,* a two-volume set published in 1923.

D. Gary Benfield, M.D.

- He wrote *Out of My Life and Thought,* an autobiography, published in 1931.
- He received honorary doctorate degrees from the University of Prague, Oxford University, St. Andrews University, the University of Chicago, and the University of Cambridge.
- In 1951, Schweitzer received a 10,000-mark prize from the West German Association of Book Publishers and Book Sellers for his efforts in promoting world peace. Schweitzer turned the money over to German refugees and destitute writers.
- A year later King Gustav Adolf awarded the Prince Charles medal to Schweitzer for his great humanitarian achievements.
- Between 1952 and 1954, Dr. Schweitzer started building a new village for Africans suffering from leprosy about a half mile from the main hospital in Lambarene. It was designed to accommodate about 250 patients.
- On October 30, 1953, he was awarded the 1952 Nobel Peace Prize. He used the money to help pay for his new leprosy hospital.
- In 1963, he celebrated the fiftieth anniversary of his hospital in Lambarene, which now consisted of 55 buildings, staffed by six physicians and 15 European nurses. Yet it still lacked enough room for patients and building still went on. Visitors came from all over the world to pay their respects and to see what he had accomplished.
- He died in Lambarene at the age of 90 on September 4, 1965, three months after I graduated from medical school.

After I bought *Out of My Life and Thought* at the Cokesbury book store, I read it from cover to cover. Deeply moved by the experience, I started thinking.

Walking the Baby Beat

If Albert Schweitzer could quit his job and get accepted to medical school at the age of 30, and spend the next seven years preparing to become a doctor, why couldn't I quit my job, go back to school, take the courses I still required for admission to medical school, get accepted to medical school, and become a doctor? If he could do it at the age of 30, why couldn't I do it at 22?

(Looking back, I'm amazed at myself. That was really me? I must have been off my rocker, or was I?)

On the other hand, my thinking was also influenced by what I knew of doctors. Growing up, I thought the doctor who removed my tonsils and the doctors who treated my sore throats were special people, possessed of special skills, as if they had been touched by the hand of God. Certainly, I wasn't anyone special, so I hadn't thought about becoming a doctor until I read these words from Schweitzer's book:

> We feel that it is not right to be permanently preoccupied with our own well-being; the welfare of others and of human society in general must become part of our responsibility.

Dr. Schweitzer had reached out and touched my heart. What should I do next?

I started hunting and gathering information. For instance, I spent an evening at the Washington Medical Center talking with an anesthesiologist about my dilemma. He was on call for the night.

He asked me why I was considering a career in medicine. In response, I stammered and stuttered, not knowing quite what to say. I said something about helping others and mentioned what I had learned from Schweitzer's example.

But he would have nothing of it. He pushed me hard, making me think. "You won't make it if it's just for others," he said. "You've got to have a selfish reason to get through it all."

As we continued talking, his phone rang. They had a 16-year-old girl in the emergency room with acute appendicitis. They were taking her to surgery and needed him to put her to sleep. He asked if I would like to come along and scrub in with him. Of course, I said yes.

He showed me how to scrub my hands, how to put on a gown, and how to stay out of the way and not touch anything within the sterile field. And during the operation, I learned something I've never forgotten: Things are not always what they seem to be.

The surgeon, a crusty old guy, made his incision and had no trouble locating the girl's appendix. But then his face got red, and he started muttering curse words under his breath. The girl's appendix was normal.

Now, any surgeon worth his salt fully expects his pre-op diagnosis to match up with what he finds at surgery. But when it doesn't, he may blow off a little steam then get back to business.

So as soon as he recovered his composure, the surgeon widened his incision and began searching for the elusive cause of his patient's symptoms. In retrospect, I think he had a pretty good idea of what he was now looking for, that's partly why he was so mad at himself.

What did he find? The girl's left fallopian tube was swollen to the size of a golf ball, indicating a tubal pregnancy. Fortunately, it hadn't ruptured. Otherwise, she might have died.

After he removed the girl's fallopian tube and was finishing up, the surgeon explained what he had done wrong:

- He hadn't asked the girl if she was sexually active, coming from a nice middle class family who were friends of his.
- He hadn't done a pelvic exam in the emergency room.
- He also hadn't done a pregnancy test before taking her to surgery.

Now he had to tell her parents, something he obviously wasn't looking forward to.

Walking the Baby Beat

I left the Washington Medical Center not fully understanding everything I had seen or heard. But as I walked across the empty parking lot and got into my car, I realized doctors are only human, like the rest of us. Perhaps I could become a doctor after all, even though I couldn't come up with a selfish reason why, even though I hadn't been touched by the hand of God.

I continued hunting and gathering information, and here's what I found:

- I was only 24 credits short of meeting the requirements to qualify for medical school.
- A residence assistant's job was open on the University of Maryland campus in College Park. It paid for room, board, and tuition for up to 10 credits a semester and four credits of summer school, just what I needed. It also paid a small stipend.

So I quit my job; sold my beloved, and almost new, tan Volkswagen car; enrolled at the University of Maryland as a special, non-degree student; and signed up for 10 credits for the fall semester of 1960. And guess what else? I landed the RA job and rejoined the marching band, playing the tuba. But I didn't stop there.

I was so naive, and so idealistic, and some might say, so dumb, that I started applying to medical schools for the following year, before the fall semester had even started. Can you believe it? And I only applied to three schools: Ohio State, Duke, and the University of Maryland.

But guess what? Sometime around Christmas, I received an invitation from the University of Maryland School of Medicine in Baltimore to interview with Dr Smith, the school's dean, and with Dr. Bradley, who headed the Department of Pediatrics.

Back then, the interviews seemed to count a lot more toward getting accepted to medical school than they do today. Now, it seems like it's more about test scores.

Both men were interested in talking about Albert Schweitzer and my idea of becoming a doctor to help others. Neither one asked me for a selfish reason for wanting to become a doctor. They also said, "Well you've got a degree in engineering, so you must know something."

So, believe it or not, I was offered a spot in the coming year's medical school class if I could pass the courses I had planned to take, and that's what I did.

Thank you, Dr. Schweitzer, for pulling me into that bookstore and showing me the way. And thank you Drs. Smith and Bradley for giving me a chance.

THE HIDDEN TALENT OF DR. SPOCK

Dr. Benjamin Spock may have arguably had a greater effect on the everyday lives of more people than any other living American. His book, *Dr. Spock's Baby and Child Care*, was revered for its down-to-earth and commonsense voice.

At the same time, in many ways, Spock was a magnet for controversy. For instance, Spock shocked his fans by protesting against the Vietnam War with Martin Luther King in 1967 and by running for president on the People's Party ticket in 1972. He was attacked by Norman Vincent Peale and Spiro Agnew for fostering a "permissive society" and by feminists for his traditional attitudes about women's role in the family.

Perhaps even more startling, however, was Spock's troubled personal life: the breakdown and alcoholism of his first wife, his own failures as husband and father, and the suicide of his grandson Peter.

But what I would like to focus on here is a hidden talent of his, a talent that helped him escape the smothering influence of his mother, Mildred, and even gain a few brief moments of respect from his otherwise indifferent father during a very special year of Spock's life.

Walking the Baby Beat

Benjamin Spock was the oldest of six children. He was born at home on May 2, 1903, in New Haven, Connecticut, in the shadow of his father's alma mater, Yale University.

His mother held strong beliefs about how to raise her children, especially the belief that her children must have lots of fresh air, no matter how cold. So each night, minutes before his father, a corporate lawyer, arrived home for dinner at seven, Mildred Spock ushered seven-year-old Benjamin and his younger siblings to the sleeping porch of their New Haven home and tucked them in for the night.

The sleeping porch rested on the second floor of the Spock's Victorian home, above the front veranda with its white picket railing. A large, striped canvas hung over the sleeping porch from a metal awning and kept away the rain and snow.

To stay warm at night in the winter, Benjamin wore Long Johns and kept a ceramic pig, warmed on the stove by his mother, beneath his heavy blankets. If the air was freezing, he put on a toboggan hat with earflaps. If he felt the urge to urinate, young Spock relieved himself in a chamber pot outside. Of course, his urine was often frozen by morning. Today, we would refer to that kind of treatment as child abuse. Back then, it might have been called disciplined child rearing.

Growing up, Mildred Spock controlled every waking minute of her oldest child's life; so much so that he didn't dare make a significant decision without discussing it first with Mother. And so, when he entered Yale University as a freshman in the fall of 1921 and his mother insisted he live at home, Benjamin reluctantly agreed.

To his fellow students then, Spock was merely a "townie," someone who didn't hang out with his pals and shoot the breeze late into the evening. Instead he went home for supper, studied alone, slept in his own bed, and grew depressed.

What pulled him out of his funk, however, was a chance encounter with the captain of the Yale rowing team who challenged Spock to go out for a man's sport. As if he had heard the voice of God, Spock walked over to the athletic office and signed up for freshman crew, without asking anyone's permission.

Spock was so far down the list of rowing team hopefuls, he was assigned to the last of 13 practice boats. Now his afternoons were consumed by crew practice in the smelly waters of New Haven Harbor.

By his sophomore year, Spock committed all his extra time to crew. "I not only wanted to be one of the boys," Spock recalled, "but I wanted to accomplish certain things. I wanted other people to recognize me as a successful striver. All of that meant an enormous amount to me, particularly against the feeling I was a mother's boy."

Spock quickly moved up the ranks, from the lowest-ranked sophomore crew, squad D, to squad A, and then to the junior varsity within one season. Clearly impressed by Ben's accomplishment, his parents finally agreed to let their son move permanently on campus.

In June 1923, all three Yale rowing teams—the varsity, freshmen, and junior varsity with Spock on board—won their races against Harvard, the first sweep for Yale against Harvard in eight years. Elated by the victory, Spock was also overwhelmed by all the hoopla: more than 25,000 people had gathered for the big event.

During his junior year, Spock moved up to the varsity and was never replaced. "As I worked up in crew, I worked out of my depression," he recalled. "My self-image was changing." And so was the Yale rowing team, which, thanks to Spock's leadership, finished its season undefeated.

The story, however, doesn't end there:

Just after final exams, the Yale rowing crew traveled to Philadelphia to compete in the 1924 Olympic trials. There they beat a heavily favored Navy crew and soon set sail for Paris to represent the United States in the 1924 Olympics.

Walking the Baby Beat

When the big race began, the Yale crew started out dead last. The big question: Could they catch up?

At an ever-increasing rate, the Yale crew's pace picked up, from 32 strokes per minute to 34, to 36 and, eventually, to a top speed of 38. By the final 500 meter mark, Yale was not only winning, but rowing away from a struggling field, beating crews from England, Italy, and Canada across the finish line.

That was heady stuff for the 6-foot, 4-inch gangly kid, known to his friends as Benny. He now had an Olympic gold medal, but, more importantly, he was now one of the boys.

The 1924 Olympic Games were remarkable for other reasons:

- In the rowing events, John B. Kelly of Philadelphia won two gold medals. His daughter, Grace, became a famous movie star and, later, the princess of Monaco.
- American Johnny Weissmuller won the gold medal in swimming. He also became a famous movie star, playing Tarzan in the movies.
- The British track-and-field team's great success later inspired the popular movie *Chariots of Fire*.

"Without a doubt, though, the Yale rowing team was most special," wrote Damon Runyon, nationally syndicated columnist at the time. "The Yale crew is America's greatest hero," continued Runyon. He even suggested that Yale University erect a marble statue with the names of Spock and his teammates inscribed on it.

Benjamin Spock went on to graduate first in his class from Columbia University's School of Medicine. He's best remembered for his pioneering book, *Dr. Spock's Baby and Child Care,* first published in 1946.

Up until the mid-1940s, parents were bombarded by experts, offering advice on how to raise their children and how to deal with their daily health needs. Even the federal government got into the act, publishing pamphlets on everything from how to prepare infant formula to how to potty train your child.

Then along came Dr. Spock, who began his new book with this truly revolutionary message for parents: "Trust yourself. You know more than you think you do."

Benjamin Spock died on March 15, 1998, at the age of 94.

Acknowledgments

The primary source for this article was Thomas Maier, *Dr. Spock: An American Life* (New York: Basic Books, 2003).

FRIEDA PUSHNIK: "THE ARMLESS AND LEGLESS WONDER"

Have you ever wondered how it is that some babies born with severe birth defects grow up and lead satisfying and very successful lives?

Well, I have, and here's what I've noticed. These children are often blessed with parents who decide early on they will not allow themselves to wallow in self-pity, and they won't allow it in their child. "If you fall down, get up and try again. If you get discouraged, I'm here to support you."

Over the years, I've seen many examples of this sort of grit and determination. Then I read about Frieda Pushnik, who topped them all.

Frieda Pushnik was born without arms or legs on February 10, 1923, in Conemaugh, Pennsylvania. From the beginning, Frieda's mother insisted she do as much as possible for herself. By holding things between a small stump of an arm and her chin, she learned to feed herself, sew, and crochet.

When Frieda was nine years old, Robert Ripley, creator of "Ripley's Believe It or Not!" heard of Frieda and arranged to visit her at home. He then asked her to appear at the World's Fair in Chicago in 1933.

Accompanied by her mother and sister, the nine-year-old joined a man who lifted weights with his eyelids and a four-year-old girl with four legs and three arms in what Ripley had named his Odditorium.

During a five-minute show repeated many times each day, she would say, "I'm Frieda Pushnik. I'm nine years old, and I attend public school." Then she would demonstrate how she could type, write, and sew. In six years of touring most of the nation's major expositions, including the New York World's Fair in 1939, she was seen by millions.

When Frieda was 20, she received a call from the Ringling Brothers and Barnum and Bailey Circus. She joined the circus's sideshow, which was in a tent pitched near the big tent's entrance and cost extra to get in.

Other attractions included giants, midgets, Siamese twins, and a tattooed man. Billed as the "Armless and Legless Wonder," she received a star's pay throughout her circus years, which lasted from 1943 to 1955.

In 1944, when the Big Top caught fire in Hartford, killing 167 people, a performer in the circus's minstrel show rushed on stage, grabbed her chair, and carried her to safety.

In the early 1960s, Frieda, her mother, her sister, and her brother-in-law moved to Orange County, California. She decorated her house with her own oil paintings, and she enjoyed entertaining. Guests, interested in watching her eat, realized after she was finished that she had been so natural they had failed to notice how she did it.

In a 1966 interview, Miss Pushnik told *The Orange County Register* that she had never resented her condition. "I never said, 'Why me?' That would be a wasted emotion. You can ruin your life like that," she said.

Frieda Pushnik died of bladder cancer on Christmas Eve 2000, at her home in Costa Mesa, California. She was 77.

Acknowledgments

Information gathered from Frieda Pushnik's obituary, which appeared in *The New York Times,* was used for this story.

D. Gary Benfield, M.D.

FRANKLIN DELANO ROOSEVELT: RESCUED AT BIRTH

When Sara Delano Roosevelt started into active labor on January 30, 1882, her doctor administered chloroform to help ease the pain. But instead, she nearly died and her baby, Franklin Delano, was limp and blue at birth. Mouth-to-mouth resuscitation and a good slap on the butt pulled the 10-pound, future President back to life.

Toward the end of labor, when a baby's head emerges from the birth canal, the birthing room fills with suspense: no one knows for sure what each baby is going to do. Fortunately, most babies breathe right away and begin crying to clear their lungs. But occasionally, even future celebrities need to be rescued from the valley of the shadow of death.

Franklin Delano Roosevelt grew up in a privileged family. He graduated from Harvard, passed the New York Bar, and married a distant cousin, Eleanor Roosevelt.

At the age of 28, he was elected to the New York State Senate, and, two years later, he was appointed Assistant Secretary of the Navy. A young man in a hurry, he was on the same political path that took his cousin Theodore Roosevelt to the White House.

But in 1921, at the age of 39, his career screeched to a halt when he was struck down by polio and paralyzed from the waist down. Roosevelt spent the next seven years in rehabilitation, determined to walk again. But he never did.

To get around, he mostly used a wheelchair. Sometimes his sons or aides carried him, or he crawled on the floor.

In 1928, Roosevelt ended his political exile and was elected governor of New York.

Four years later, he was elected to the first of four consecutive terms as president of the United States.

After guiding this country through the Great Depression and through most of World War II, Roosevelt suffered a stroke and died in 1945.

Walking the Baby Beat

In 1995, Senate Majority Leader Robert Dole made a speech on the floor of the U.S. Senate to honor the 50th anniversary of FDR's death. In that speech Dole referred to Roosevelt as a disability hero. But it was not because FDR had displayed courage and grit in the face of overwhelming odds. It was because of his efforts on behalf of others with disabilities.

In 1926, while still in rehabilitation from his bout with polio, Roosevelt purchased a run-down resort in Warm Springs, Georgia. And over the next 20 years he turned it into a unique, first-class rehabilitation center.

The center's approach was based on a new philosophy of treatment—one where psychological recovery was as important as medical treatment.

FDR believed in an independent life for people with disabilities at a time when society thought they should be tucked away in the closet.

Warm Springs was run by people with polio, for people with polio. In that spirit, Roosevelt was the father of the modern independent living movement, which puts people with disabilities in control of their own lives.

Sometimes a little mouth-to-mouth and a good slap on the butt works wonders.

DR. IGNAZ SEMMELWEIS: "YOU MUST WASH YOUR HANDS!"

What's the most effective way to prevent the spread of infectious diseases? If you answered good hand washing, you're correct. But few people, including most doctors, associate good hand washing with an obscure obstetrician named Ignaz Semmelweis, who practiced in Vienna more than 150 years ago.

Now, without reading another word, you might be asking yourself, "Why is Semmelweis one of his heroes? The man's name is hard to pronounce, and he died more than 100 years ago. What did he accomplish that was so noble?"

For the answer, you'll have to read on. But I will give you a hint: At a time of great ignorance about infectious diseases, Semmelweis, an outsider to Vienna from Hungary, made several discoveries that saved hundreds of lives, but could have saved thousands more had the doctors of Vienna listened to him. Why didn't they listen? In part because they would have had to admit to themselves that they had caused thousands upon thousands of women throughout Europe to die of childbed fever, simply because they had refused to wash their hands.

Ignaz Philipp Semmelweis was born in Hungary on July 1, 1818, the fifth child of a successful merchant. While growing up, he had blond hair, blue-gray eyes, and an easy smile. As a young man, he was described as lighthearted, popular, and a bit on the heavy side. But, after he finished medical school and found a job at the Vienna General Hospital, his personality would change dramatically.

In February 1846, at the age of 28, Semmelweis started to work as first assistant in obstetrics at the Vienna General Hospital, home to the world's largest birthing center. His job included teaching medical students, assisting with surgical procedures, and taking responsibility for the patients' care.

The obstetrics service was divided into two divisions. The first division, which he was responsible for, was for training medical students in obstetrics while the second division was for training midwives. Women in labor were admitted to the first division on Mondays, Wednesdays, and Fridays. Otherwise, they were admitted to the second division on Tuesdays, Thursdays, and over the weekends.

At the end of Semmelweis's first month on the job, he was stunned to find that 17 percent of mothers on the first division had died of childbed fever after giving birth. Also known as puerperal fever, Semmelweis had no first-hand knowledge about the disease. However, he had been taught in medical school that puerperal fever was merely an unfortunate and unavoidable part of childbirth, caused by, among other things, bad air. That explanation hadn't phased him while a medical student, but now that he had met these women and had been their doctor, he was deeply disturbed and set out to try and understand this mysterious disease.

During the ensuing year, Semmelweis kept close tabs on the maternal mortality rates for both divisions. Again, he was stunned by what he learned: Roughly 10 percent of the mothers who delivered on the first division had died from childbed fever after giving birth while less than 1 percent of the mothers who delivered on the second division had met the same fate.

He was also disturbed to learn that the high death toll on the first division was well known by the lower class women of Vienna, who normally delivered there. They desperately sought to avoid being admitted on Mondays, Wednesdays, or Fridays, preferring instead to deliver in a doorway or back alley. On the other hand, women of means gave birth at home and were relatively free of the dreaded disease.

Semmelweis reasoned that because the two divisions were side by side in the same building, if childbed fever was genuinely an epidemic disease then the number of cases should be roughly the same in both divisions.

He also couldn't understand why anyone could go on thinking that childbed fever was an unfortunate and unavoidable part of childbirth that struck most often on certain days of the week

Why, he wondered, was the difference so striking? So he drew up several comparisons between the two divisions:

- In both divisions of the hospital, the physical conditions were the same; in fact, conditions were worse in the second division because it was always overcrowded.
- Midwives delivered their patients while lying on their side, so Semmelweis adopted the same procedure, but nothing changed.

- When it was suggested that midwives were more gentle than medical students or physicians, Semmelweis practiced the greatest possible gentleness without effect.
- All the textbooks mentioned fear as one of the causes of childbed fever. Semmelweis noticed that the hospital priest always passed through the first division, ringing a bell as he walked on the way to the chapel, so Semmelweis asked him not to ring the bell as he came through. But nothing changed.

Desperate to find an answer, Semmelweis started each day by meeting his medical students in the morgue, where they performed autopsies on the women who had died from childbed fever. During the course of each autopsy, the organs were removed from the body and passed around for each student to touch and see. What they found was always the same: pus and inflammation throughout the body.

At the time, remember, there was no sterile technique, cleansing of instruments, or routine hand washing. Doctors wore their street clothes when they operated in surgery, delivered a baby, saw patients in their office, or performed an autopsy in the morgue. So, during the course of a typical working day, a doctor simply wiped his hands on his clothes to clean them. (Thirty more years would pass before Pasteur discovered that bacteria carried on the hands can cause infectious diseases.)

After completing their dissections, Semmelweis and his students went directly to the maternity ward where they carefully performed pelvic exams on their patients. All the while, their clothes and hands reeked of pus from the autopsy room.

Semmelweis finally got the break he needed in March 1847 when a pathologist friend, Dr. Kolletschka, died from an infected scalpel wound, accidentally inflicted by a medical student during an autopsy on one of the childbed fever cases. The autopsy report on Kolletschka revealed pus and inflammation throughout his body, the same exact findings as those typically found in women who died from childbed fever and some of their infants.

After reviewing the autopsy report, Semmelweis made up a list of terrifying assumptions:

- What if the knife had introduced cadaverous material into Kollectschka's wound, causing an infection that spread throughout his body and killed him?
- Had he and his students introduced the same deadly material into the birth canals of his patients after they had carried it on their hands from the autopsy room to the labor and delivery area?
- This reasoning would also explain why the maternal death rate on the second division was so low: The midwives never went to the autopsy room.
- This reasoning would also explain why first-time mothers were more prone to the disease. Because their labors lasted longer, he and his students examined them more often than women who delivered quickly.
- If his list of assumptions was correct, he now had an explanation for a cause of childbed fever and for the differences between the maternal death rates on the two divisions.

Grief stricken by the implications of his horrifying thoughts, Semmelweis took his concerns to the head of Obstetrics, Professor Klein, but he didn't seem to care. Meanwhile, the medical students were apathetic, and the nurses were indifferent, all of which added to his frustration.

So Semmelweis pulled himself together and set out to test his idea. On May 15, 1847, he posted the following notice on the clinic door:

> As of today, every doctor or student who comes from the dissecting room is required, before entering the maternity

wards, to wash his hands thoroughly in a basin of chlorine water which is being placed at the entrance. This order applies to all without exception.

Initially, the response to Semmelweis's basin of chlorine water was mixed: some physicians and medical students did as requested while others found it too troublesome to wash their hands. So Semmelweis had to stand guard by the basin and force everyone to wash their hands. As a result, the number of maternal deaths in the first division, during the next few months, dropped dramatically to 3 percent, the lowest it had ever been.

But on October 2, 1847, just when Semmelweis was starting to feel good about his accomplishment, he discovered 12 women deathly ill from childbed fever on his ward. Even though 9 of the 12 eventually died, he didn't give up. He investigated each case, grew more obsessed than ever, and found a common thread.

Semmelweis and his students had washed their hands before examining a woman with uterine cancer. Then they had moved on and examined the other patients without washing their hands between patients. Semmelweis now reasoned that infectious materials could be carried not only from the dead to the living, but from diseased living patients to other healthy patients.

With this new discovery, Semmelweis ordered the following additions to his program of hand washing:

- Stringent hand washing was ordered before every exam.
- Semmelweis supervised the cleaning of all instruments that he, like all doctors, had previously wiped off on their coattails.
- Sick maternity patients with inflamed or discharging wounds were placed in isolation rooms.

In 1848, the first full year after Semmelweis had expanded his program of hand washing, the maternal mortality rate in the first division hit an all-time low: 1.27 percent compared with 1.33 percent in the second division. But, behind his back, students, nurses, and other physicians complained bitterly to Professor Klein, who vowed to rid himself of the fanatical troublemaker at the first opportunity.

Semmelweis had no idea that bacteria were the cause of childbed fever and all other surgical fevers, a discovery that lay 30 years ahead. But he identified the route by which doctors were transmitting the disease, a concept that would eventually form the basis for aseptic techniques.

Semmelweis was repeatedly urged by two of his friends, Drs. Skoda and Hebra, to write a paper about his discoveries and submit it for publication in a medical journal. At first, he hesitated because he felt awkward expressing himself in writing. But then he was offered the chance to present a series of lectures on his discoveries before the Vienna Medical Society. He hoped those lectures would satisfy even the most hardened of his critics and bring them over to his way of thinking.

But before Semmelweis was scheduled to present the lectures, his contract in the Department of Obstetrics at the Vienna General Hospital came up for renewal. And guess what? Professor Klein refused to renew it, costing Semmelweis his job.

Now out of work, Semmelweis had plenty of time to prepare his lectures, which he presented to high praise on three occasions during 1850. At this point, the Semmelweis theory of puerperal fever stood on the verge of acceptance, even though he was out of work. It had the support of the emerging leaders of Vienna medicine, and Semmelweis had capably defended himself in an open forum. All he now had to do was write up his lectures, submit them for publication, and gain final acceptance. But nothing could persuade him to write.

Still unable to find a job in Vienna that was satisfactory and outraged by the knowledge that thousands of women throughout Europe were dying needlessly, Semmelweis abruptly left Vienna. Without saying a word to his friends, he returned to Hungary, where he slipped into seclusion.

Meanwhile, in Vienna no one spoke of Semmelweis any longer. His successor at the Vienna General Hospital abolished Semmelweis's basins of chlorine water and his expanded program of hand washing, and returned to the old ways of doing things.

A year later, early in 1851, Semmelweis was invited by a surgeon friend in Budapest to visit the maternity ward at Saint Roche's Hospital. There Semmelweis found six mothers, who had just delivered, dying of childbed fever. Their doctor routinely went back and forth between his patients on the surgical ward, with their festering wounds, and the maternity cases on the obstetrics ward without washing his hands, cleaning his instruments, or changing clothes.

Believing he could still make a difference, Semmelweis applied for the unfilled job of head of the maternity division at St. Roche's. But he had to swallow his pride and settle for the unpaid position as honorary chief of the section in May 1851.

Far from Vienna and the world of science, Semmelweis started over again. Once more he placed basins of chlorine water in strategic places. Once more he insisted that everyone wash their hands, between each patient exam and after leaving the morgue. And, of course, he encountered resistance and scorn, but he persisted.

Over the next six years he reduced the maternal morality rate from childbed fever at St. Roche's to less than 1 percent while, at this time, the maternal mortality rate in Vienna was still between 10 and 15 percent. He also learned something new: unclean bed linens could transmit infectious materials and cause disease. As a result, he won a hard fought battle to have the bed linens changed and laundered on a regular basis.

During this period, Semmelweis married and started a family. He also built a large private practice. And, believe it or not, the Hungarian government officially endorsed his methods.

Walking the Baby Beat

Finally, hoping to set the record straight, he decided to write a book about childbed fever. Published in 1861, parts of the book included factual and moving accounts of his discoveries while, in other parts, he lashed out against his critics, calling them murderers and other names, which did not help his cause.

Semmelweis assumed that his book would mark a turning point in the acceptance of his discoveries. Not only was he wrong, but the book actually worsened his position. Now his opponents had a highly visible target against which to launch their assaults, and they did. At a conference of German physicians and natural scientists, most of the speakers rejected his ideas. And when Rudolph Virchow, later known as the father of modern pathology, opposed his ideas, few people took Semmelweis seriously anymore. He became living proof of the Hungarian proverb: "Tell the truth, and people will bash in your head."

Exasperated and depressed, Semmelweis lashed out at his critics, both publicly and in private, accusing them of arrogance in the face of truth and repeatedly calling them murderers. Then, over the next four years his mental health deteriorated rapidly.

Overwhelmed by the medical community's callous indifference and by the knowledge that innocent women would go on dying from childbed fever, Semmelweis lost all touch with reality.

Finally, in July 1865, at the age of 47, his wife admitted him to an insane asylum where he died a few weeks later. Legend has it that the autopsy on his body revealed a familiar picture: pus and inflammation throughout his body. During one of his last deliveries, Semmelweis had cut his finger. The very disease he had devoted his professional life to fighting had entered through the wound.

However, after extensive research, Sherwin B. Nuland, M.D., emeritus professor of surgery at Yale University, published a different ending to Semmelweis's life. Yes, after several years of rapid aging and mental deterioration, his wife was forced to have him committed to a public asylum in Vienna. But, there he became violent and was beaten by asylum personnel, dying a short time later from the injuries he received. The myth that he had died in a manner befitting a Greek tragedy no longer holds true.

Years later, when Pasteur discovered that the pus and inflammation Semmelweis found at the many autopsies he conducted was caused by bacteria carried on the hands, the medical world finally accepted the significance of Semmelweis's contributions. As a result, the Medical University of Budapest, where he worked, was named after him and he received wide acclaim, though now dead.

A further thought: Henrik Ibsen's famous play, "An Enemy of the People" (1882), is the dramatic story of a doctor whose work and fate are loosely modeled after the tragedy of Ignaz Semmelweis. Dr. Stockman, a simple country doctor, tries to protect the people from using the town spa, which is contaminated with pathogenic bacteria. His discovery, however, conflicts with people's belief in the therapeutic properties of their treasured spa and jeopardizes the town's economy, which relies heavily on the tourist trade. The city's leaders and the public both denounce Dr. Stockman as "an enemy of the people."

DR. MARTIN A. COUNEY: THE "INCUBATOR-BABY DOCTOR"

On Thursday morning, March 2, 1950, the following obituary appeared in *The New York Times:*

> Dr. Martin A. Couney, a specialist in the care of prematurely born infants, who had shown such babies to the public for an admission price at fairs and other exhibitions throughout the United States and in Europe for more than fifty years, died last night at his home, 3728 Surf Avenue, Coney Island. He was 80 years old.

Walking the Baby Beat

"The Incubator Doctor," as Dr. Couney was informally known, was born in Germany, studied medicine in Breslau, Berlin, and Leipzig, receiving an M.D., and later in Paris under Dr. Pierre C. Budin, noted pediatrician, who developed a method of saving the prematurely born.

At the Berlin Exposition in 1896, Dr. Couney operated an exhibit of prematurely born babies to show the Budin technique. The exhibit was a financial success, as was a second one at Earl's Court in London.

In 1898 Dr. Couney paid his first visit to the United States and staged an exhibit at the Omaha Trans-Mississippi Exposition. He returned to Paris for the exposition of 1900, but was back in this country for the Buffalo Exposition the next year, and then decided to remain here for good.

For years he had shows at both Dreamland and Luna Park, and the night Dreamland was destroyed by fire the babies were saved by a quick transfer to the Luna Park incubators, some of the lodgers doubling up.

Dr. Couney had one of his Baby incubator attractions at the New York World's Fair (1939–1940). He leaves a daughter, Hildegarde Couney, long associated with her father's affairs. His wife, Annabelle May Couney, died in 1938.

After reading Dr. Couney's obituary, one might say, "What a bizzare man!"

Dr. Couney was a showman, no doubt about that. But don't be fooled. His Coney Island incubator baby exhibit provided state-of-the-art care for premature babies and saved many lives for many years. No hospital in the United States could match it.

In the 1890s, France led the world in premature baby care, thanks to two hospitals in Paris, the Paris Maternity Hospital and the Clinique Tarnier. They were the first centers in the world to create premature nurseries for the care and study of "weaklings."

Directed by Dr. Pierre Budin (pronounced *boo-dan*), a highly respected pediatrician, both nurseries featured the following:

- Highly skilled wet nurses who provided breast milk and bedside care.
- Incubators modeled after the warming chambers used for rearing poultry at the Paris Zoo.
- The technique of gavage or tube feeding, used when a preemie was too immature to suck and swallow effectively.

In comparison, hospital care for premature infants didn't begin in the United States until the 1920s when Dr. Julius Hess opened the premature baby care unit at Michael Reese Hospital in Chicago.

Even though France was the world leader in premature baby care, Dr. Budin lacked a stamp of approval from the German scientific community. So what did he do? He decided to dispatch his young assistant, Dr. Martin Couney, to the Berlin Exposition of 1896 to exhibit six of his latest incubators.

But Couney had his own ideas. Why not take along an entourage of Dr. Budin's wet nurses, fill the incubators with live preemies, and name the exhibit "Kinderbrutanstalt" or the Child Hatchery?

After obtaining Dr. Budin's approval, Couney contacted the Empress Augusta Victoria, benefactor for Berlin's Charity Hospital, who agreed to supply the needed babies. After all, they weren't expected to survive anyway.

The notion of a "child hatchery" caught on with the Berlin public. Soon crude songs about the exhibit were heard in the beer halls and night clubs. Located in the amusement section next to the Congo Village and the Tyrolean Yodelers, it was a huge success, always jammed with people willing to pay a mark to see the delightful "little birds."

The German scientific community was equally impressed; "there were no deaths," according to Couney, who returned home with a handsome profit in his pocket.

The following year, Couney was asked to repeat his performance, this time in London.

Walking the Baby Beat

At the last minute, London physicians refused to refer their preemies to Couney for care.

So what do you suppose Dr. Couney did?

He wired Dr. Budin about his plight and asked for help. In response, Budin shipped six Paris preemies in wicker baskets across the English Channel and saved the show. It turned out to be a big hit, not only with the British public, but, eventually, the British medical community as well.

After a successful taste of show business, Dr. Martin Couney immigrated to America in 1903 and set up an incubator baby exhibit on the midway at Coney Island. The sign above the entrance read, "Everybody Loves a Baby."

Couney exhibited there from spring to fall for the next 40 years. He also married Annabelle May, an Irish nurse, who was an expert in premature baby care.

Each spring, Couney hired four or five wet nurses to supply his patients with milk until the exhibit closed in the fall. To maintain their milk production, Couney's nursing staff hired out on private cases during the winter and returned the following spring.

Recognizing the need to maintain morale, he offered weekly prizes of nylon stockings to the nurse whose babies had gained the most weight.

Couney's daughter, Hildegarde, was born prematurely in midwinter, forcing her father to open the exhibition building, where she spent the first three months of her life in an incubator. After she grew up, she became a nurse and worked with her father.

In addition to the annual shows at Coney Island, Couney exhibited in other parts of the world:

- Portland, Oregon, in 1906
- Mexico City in 1908
- Rio de Janiero in 1910
- Denver, Colorado, in 1913
- And periodically in Atlantic City and in Chicago

In all his shows, Couney was proud of the fact that he never took a cent from the parents. In addition, parents received free passes to view their babies just like other paying customers. However, they were not allowed to participate in their babies' care until the day of discharge. Little wonder then that some parents were reluctant to take their babies home.

In 1933–1934, at the Chicago's Century of Progress Exposition, Couney's exhibit was located on the midway next to Sally Rand's show. The famous fan dancer often complained to police officers, when they came to arrest her for indecent exposure, that Couney's babies wore fewer clothes than she did, yet no one said a thing about them.

Couney enjoyed a good reputation among the obstetricians in the New York area. They sent infants to his exhibit confident that the babies would receive skilled care. In 1937, he was honored by New York's Medical Society and presented with a platinum watch.

The infant incubator exhibit was Coney Island's oddest and, at times, most popular attraction. The 25 cent admission fee also payed for the development of ground-breaking technology far more sophisticated than any available in most hospitals. The survival rate was unsurpassed by any medical facility in the world.

The 1939–1940 New York World's Fair was financially difficult for Couney because viewing premature babies was becoming old hat to the public. So when the first premature nursery opened in New York City in the early 1940's, Couney closed his Coney Island show for good.

A pioneering pediatrician and showman, who became known as the Incubator-Baby Doctor, Martin Couney was the first doctor in the United States to offer infants such specialized care.

A further thought: An aspiring actor named Archibald Leach worked as a barker for Couney's sideshow while waiting for a part in an upcoming Broadway musical. He went on to become a famous movie idol under the name given him by Paramount Pictures: Cary Grant.

Acknowledgment

A primary source for this article was Dr. William A. Silverman, "Incubator-Baby Side Shows," *Pediatrics* (August 1979).

SUDDENLY PARAPLEGIC, JOSEPH STOCK NEVER GAVE UP

Each week, the *Journal of the American Medical Association* displays a work of fine art on its cover. In June 2001, the *JAMA* featured "Baby in Wicker Basket" by Joseph Whiting Stock (1815–1855).

Joseph Stock was born on January 30, 1815, in Springfield, Massachusetts. Months before, the British had captured Washington, D.C., and burned the Capitol and the White House. But when the British fleet bombarded Fort McHenry in Baltimore harbor, they were turned back. During the battle, Francis Scott Key wrote the lyrics to "The Star Spangled Banner," our national anthem.

In 1826, at the age of 11, an oxcart fell on young Stock, paralyzing him from the waist down. Unable to sit, and lying almost constantly in one position, he remained in his room for almost six years.

But when Stock was 17, his family's physician introduced him to Franklin White, a local artist. Wanting to learn how to do something useful, Stock began studying painting with White.

At the age of 19—and now bedridden for eight years—Stock was commissioned by Dr. Joseph Swain to do a series of anatomical drawings. But more importantly, the doctor designed and constructed a wheelchair which enabled the artist to sit up and move about his parents' home. Before long, Stock was able to travel by train and work like any other artist.

D. Gary Benfield, M.D.

Tragedy struck again on New Year's Day 1939. Stock was severely burned about the face and hands in a fire that occurred when he was making varnishes for his paintings. Less than three weeks later, Stock, according to Dr. Swain, was struck by congestive typhus, which left him partially deranged at times.

This incident was followed by a severe pressure sore that gradually ate away at his right hip joint. Then, just when hope for recovery had all but vanished, Dr. Swain consulted a colleague who operated and removed the head of Stock's damaged femur. Despite a long recovery, Stock produced the bulk of his work in the remaining years of his life.

"Baby in Wicker Basket" is typical of the many children's portraits Stock painted. It features a cheruby-cheeked, chin-dimpled child holding a favorite rattle against the background of a patterned rug.

It was a common practice at the time for parents to order a portrait of a child who had died. The artist often had nothing more to work with than a parent's description or an assortment of the child's belongings. It was also customary for young children, boys and girls alike, to wear dresses.

Stock died of tuberculosis at the age of 40, in the city where he was born. Though his life was tragically short and filled with difficulties, Stock sold more than 900 paintings between 1832 and 1846. More than 100 additional paintings remained in his studio at the time of his death.

Stock's work lives on a century and a half after his death, thanks to a physician's interest and skill, and to the fortitude and talent of a young man who would not give up. Three of his paintings are in the National Gallery of Art's permanent collection. They can be seen on the Gallery's Web site, www.nga.gov.

Resource Center

PLANNING YOUR PREGNANCY

1. "Are You Ready? A Guide to Planning A Healthy, Happy Pregnancy"
   Planning to have a baby? Just thinking about it? This 48-page booklet from the March of Dimes may be right for you.
   Booklet available in English or Spanish.
   Price: $22.50/pkg of 10
   To order online, go to www.marchofdimes.com.
   To order by phone, call the March of Dimes Fulfillment Center at 800-367-6630.

2. "Think Ahead for a Healthy Baby"
   This pamphlet offers 10 simple steps a woman can take before pregnancy to prepare for the birth of a healthy baby. Includes tips on taking folic acid, the risks of drinking alcohol, smoking, and drugs, and the importance of a pre-pregnancy checkup.
   Pamphlet available in English or Spanish
   Price: $22.50/pkg of 10
   To order online, go to www.marchofdimes.com.
   To order by phone, call the March of Dimes Fulfillment Center at 800-367-6630.

PREGNANCY

1. *Mayo Clinic Guide to a Healthy Pregnancy*
   Editor in Chief: Roger Harms, M.D.
   This new Mayo Clinic book provides you with practical information and reassurance about the exciting

and sometimes unpredictable journey through pregnancy and childbirth.
Published by Harper Collins
Price: Approx. $19.95

2. *Your Pregnancy Week by Week*
   Authors: Glade B. Curtis, M.D., and Judith Schuler, M.S.
   Pregnant women will especially like the week-by-week format of this best-selling book.
   Published by Da Capo Life Long, a member of the Perseus Books Group
   Price: $15.95
   469 pages

Note: Glade B. Curtis, M.D., and Judith Schuler, M.S. have also published these books:
   Your Baby's First Year
   Your Pregnancy Questions and Answers
   Your Pregnancy for the Father-to-Be
   Your Pregnancy Journal Week by Week
   Bouncing Back After Your Pregnancy
   Your Pregnancy—Every Woman's Guide
   Your Pregnancy After 35

PREMATURE BIRTH

1. *The Premature Baby Book: Everything You Need To Know About Your Premature Baby From Birth to Age One*
   Authors: Dr. William Sears and family
   If your baby is born prematurely, it's natural to feel special concern. In the first few weeks after your baby's birth, you may grapple not only with complex medical decisions but also with the need to anticipate developmental issues that could affect your child later on. *The Premature Baby Book* offers

the tools and advice you need to become comfortable with a potentially bewildering new role.
Published by Little Brown and Co.
Price: 15.95
244 pages

Note: Dr. William Sears and his family have also published these books:
The Baby Book
The Pregnancy Book
The Attachment Parenting Book
The Breastfeeding Book
The Fussy Baby Book
The Discipline Book
The Family Nutrition Book
The Successful Child

2. Parenting Your Premature Baby and Child: The Emotional Journey
Authors: Deborah L. Davis, Ph.D and Mara Tesler Stein, Psy. D.

Many good books explain your premature baby's medical or developmental conditions and treatments, and guide you in caregiving tasks. This book is different. It focuses on your experiences, feelings, and relationships around the delivery, hospitalization, homecoming, and long-term parenting of your premature baby and child. It provides suggestions and support for coping, adjusting, and finding your way.
Published by Fulcrum Publishing
Price: $24.95
901 pages

3. American Association for Premature Infants
This organization engages in advocacy, and offers a newsletter and other resources.
Cincinnati, Ohio
513-522-8040
www.aapi-online.org

4. Clothing and Accessories for Preemies
   www.earlybirds.com
   www.preemie.com
   www.tinybundles.com

BREASTFEEDING

1. *The Womanly Art of Breastfeeding,* 7th edition
   Author: La Leche League International
       First published in 1958, this classic guide to breastfeeding is filled with the results of current research along with personal stories from mothers. The seventh revised edition offers new explanations of how the breast makes milk, details about effective positioning and latch-on, suggestions for using herbs and medications to increase milk supply, and more.
   Published by the Penguin Group
   Price: $16.95
   480 pages
       You can purchase this book at your local bookstore or from the La Leche League International online bookstore at www.lalecheleague.org.

2. *Defining Your Own Success: Breastfeeding after Breast Reduction Surgery*
   Author: Diana West
       This first-of-a-kind book addresses the questions and myths associated with if and how a mother can breastfeed after breast reduction surgery. It combines up-to-date research with experience and advice from breastfeeding mothers who have had breast reduction surgery.
   328 pages
   Price: Approx.$18.50
       You can purchase this book at your local bookstore or from the La Leche League International online bookstore at www.lalecheleague.org.

3. *Breastfeeding Your Premature Baby,* Revised Edition
   Author: Gwen Gotsch
   This La Leche League International book offers clear and concise information about how to breastfeed your premature baby and why breastfeeding is important for your baby. In addition to breast feeding basics, the book offers complete information on pumping, storing your milk, how to use nipple shields, and how to position your baby correctly at the breast, supporting both neck and shoulders.
   56 pages
   Price: Approx. $5.95
   You can purchase this book at your local bookstore or from the La Leche League International online bookstore at www.lalecheleague.org.

4. *The Breastfeeding Book: Everything You Need to Know About Nursing Your Child from Birth Through Weaning*
   Authors: Martha Sears, R.N., and William Sears, M.D.
   Martha Sears nursed all eight of her children, so she has plenty of experience to share with her readers. Some women, however, have been a bit turned off by the section devoted to women trying to decide whether to return to work and how their decision might affect their ability to continue breastfeeding. Overall, it is an excellent book with an obvious bias in places that may seem, to some women, as slightly condescending.
   Publisher: Little, Brown
   Price: Varies around $14.95
   272 pages

BABY AND CHILD CARE

1. *Caring for Your Baby and Young Child: Birth to Age 5*
   Editor-in-Chief: Steven P. Shelov, M.D.
   This comprehensive book, one of a series of three, offers state-of-the-art advice for mothers,

fathers, and caregivers from the American Academy of Pediatrics.
Published by the American Academy of Pediatrics (AAP)
Price: Approx. $17.95 in soft cover
701 pages
   You can purchase this book at your local bookstore or from the AAP online bookstore at www.aap.org/bookstore.

2. *Caring for Your School-Age Child: Ages 5 to 12*
Editor-in-Chief: Edward L. Schor, M.D.
   This comprehensive book, number two in a series of three, also offers state-of-the-art advice for mothers, fathers, and caregivers from the American Academy of Pediatrics.
Published by the American Academy of Pediatrics
Price: Approx. $29.95 in hard cover
596 pages
   You can purchase this book at your local bookstore or from the AAP online bookstore at www.aap.org/bookstore.

3. *Caring for Your Adolescent: Ages 12 to 21*
Editor-in-Chief: Donald E. Greydanus, M.D.
   This comprehensive book, the third in this series, also offers state-of-the-art advice for mothers, fathers, and caregivers from the American Academy of Pediatrics.
Published by the American Academy of Pediatrics
Price: Approx. $24.50 in hard cover
326 pages
   You can purchase this book at your local bookstore or from the AAP online bookstore at www.aap.org/bookstore.

Walking the Baby Beat

4. *Heading Home with Your Newborn: From Birth to Reality*
   Authors: Laura A. Jana, M.D. and Jennifer Shu, M.D.

   "As entertaining as it is authoritative: a warm, witty, sensible, and solid contribution to parenting . . . parents will love this book."
   —Robert Needlman, M.D., coauthor, *Dr. Spock's Baby and Child Care*.

   Published by the American Academy of Pediatrics
   Price: $14.95
   306 pages
   You can purchase this book at your local bookstore or from the AAP online bookstore at www.aap.org/bookstore.

5. *Dr. Spock's Baby and Child Care: A Handbook for Parents of Developing Children from Birth Through Adolescence*
   Authors: Benjamin Spock, M.D. (now deceased) and Robert Needlman, M.D.

   When this timeless bestseller was first published by Dr. Spock back in the 1940s, it opened with this advice to parents: "Trust yourself. You know more than you think you do." Now in its eighth edition, the book has been revised and updated many times, but Dr. Spock's #1 rule of parenting has remained the same: "Trust yourself. You know more than you think you do."
   Published by Pocket Books
   Price: Approx. $18.00
   967 pages

6. *Touchpoints: Your Child's Emotional and Behavioral Development*
   Author: T. Berry Brazelton, M.D.

351

D. Gary Benfield, M.D.

"Touchpoints" are the spurts of development and the trying periods of regression that every child goes through during childhood. In this best-selling book, Dr. Brazelton uses these touchpoints to help parents understand their child's behavior and to prevent future problems.
Published by Addison-Wesley Publishing Company
Price: Approx. $16.00
469 pages

TWINS AND HIGHER MULTIPLES

1. *Having Twins and More: A Parent's Guide to Multiple Pregnancy, Birth, and Early Childhood*
   Authors: Elizabeth Noble with Leo Sorger, M.D.
   When the first edition of this best-selling book hit the bookstores back in 1980, it was one of the first, if not the first book on twins and higher multiples. Now in its third edition, this book remains a valuable contribution to the resources parents of multiples have available to them.
   Houghton Mifflin Co.
   Price: $18.95
   560 pages

2. National Organization of Mothers of Twins Clubs
   (877) 540-2200 or (615) 595-0936
   www.nomotc.org

3. *Twins Magazine*
   A national magazine that focuses on topics related to multiples.
   www.twinsmagazine.com

GENETICS AND BIRTH DEFECTS

1. *Your Genetic Destiny: Know Your Genes, Secure Your Health, Save Your Life*
   Author: Aubrey Milunsky, M.D., D.Sc.
      This book is an authoritative guide to the risks of genetic disorders and life-saving information for you and your family.

   "Fascinating, easy to read . . . a valuable contribution. A practitioner would be doing his patient and future generations an important service by calling attention to this book."
   —*The New York Times*

   Published by Perseus Publishing
   Price: Approx. $27.50
   410 pages

2. The March of Dimes Web site: www.marchofdimes.com
      Looking for information about genetics and birth defects? You'll find answers to many of your questions here. This site is also worth bookmarking for future use. You can check out the March of Dimes product catalog for items you may want to buy online.

PERINATAL LOSS

1. The Compassionate Friends
      This nondenominational self-help organization offers support and friendship to families following the death of a child. Its mission is to assist families toward the positive resolution of grief following the

D. Gary Benfield, M.D.

death of a child of any age and to provide information to help others be supportive. Through its affiliation with Centering Corporation, Your Grief Resource Center, The Compassionate Friends offers more than 400 grief resources for children and adults. The Web site address is www.compassionatefriends.org.

The organization includes more than 500 chapters worldwide.

The Compassionate Friends
P.O. Box 3696
Oak Brook, IL 60522
(877)-969-0010

2. The March of Dimes Web site:
www.marchofdimes.com
The March of Dimes offers a variety of helpful materials about perinatal loss on its Web site, including the following:

- An extensive listing if support groups for parents and grandparents who have experienced a miscarriage, stillbirth, newborn loss, or the loss of an older child
- Extensive fact sheets about each of these types of losses
- Bereavement materials, including a March of Dimes Bereavement Kit

Parents or other family members who have experienced the loss of a baby between conception and the first month of life can receive a free Bereavement Kit by completing the online order form. To order by phone, call the March of Dimes Fulfillment Center at 800-367-6630

3. *Motherhood & Mourning Perinatal Death*
Authors: Larry G. Peppers and Ronald J. Knapp

Walking the Baby Beat

This widely proclaimed book provides grieving mothers with an understanding of the grief process and the attitudes toward infant death in our society. As a result, it helps them to realize they are not alone: Other women share the same problems. Although the book was published in 1980, it is still available new, at least through Amazon.com. However the asking price is awfully steep at $93.00. If it were my money, I would buy a used copy through Amazon.com for under $10.00.
Published by Praeger Special Studies
Price: $93.00 new; less than $10.00 used
165 pages

Index

A

abducted and missing children
  killers, profile of, 226
  nonfamily abduction, 225–226
  photo cards sent in mail,
    effectiveness of, 228
  preventing, guide for parents, 227–228
  runaway *vs.* thrownaway child, 224–225
  sexual assault, 225, 226
Accutane, 2, 14–15
acetaminophen, 160, 188, 242
acne, and Accutane, 2, 14–15
African Americans
  breastfeeding, 112
  head lice, 259
  mongolian spots, 209–210, 211
  sickle cell disease, 2, 90–91
  sun protection, 242–243
Agnew, Spiro, 322
AIDS, 22–23
Akron Children's Hospital
  Annual Remembrance Service, 244–245
  Genetics Center, 94
  neonatal intensive care unit, 65
Alaya, Abraham, 290
Alaya, Airon, 289
Alaya, Anissa, 289–290
Alaya, Marissa-Eve, 290
Alaya, Mary, 289–290
alcohol consumption
  coffee drinking and, 113
  during pregnancy, 2
  by teens, 228, 262–263, 287
allergies
  to antibiotics, 194–195
  to food, 135
  rhinitis, 206
Alzheimer's disease, 89, 297
American Academy of Pediatrics (AAP)
  on amoxicillin, and breast milk, 103
  on caffeine consumption, 21
  on chickenpox vaccine,
    recommended dose, 198, 202
  on choking, in infants, 154
  on circumcision, 72–74
  on cough suppressants, 205
  on CPR classes, 154
  on DEET-containing products, 203
  on ear infections, treatment of, 200
  on excluding children from daycare
    due to illness, 232–233
  on fluoride for babies, 167
  on genitals, toddler's discovery of and
    parent's response to, 182
  on head lice, 256–258, 259
  on Lithium, and breast milk, 9, 103
  on obesity in children, 275
  Pediatrics medical journal, 52, 53,
    200, 236, 343
  on poison ivy treatment, 213–214
  on propanalol, and breast milk, 105
  on Prozac, and breast milk, 114
  on reading crisis, 148
  reference resources from, 350–351
  on shaken baby syndrome, temper
    control in caregivers, 234
  on SIDS prevention guidelines ("Back
    to Sleep" campaign), 121–123,
    124, 125
  on sports participation, medical
    conditions affecting, 261
  on television viewing, of children
    under age two, 184–185
  Virginia Apgar postage stamp
    campaign participation, 314
  on vitamin K supplement for
    newborns, 119
  on vitamin supplements, for healthy
    babies, 163
  on walkers for babies, 221
  on water births, 52–53
American Heart Association, CPR
  classes, 154, 289
American Herbal Products Association, 21
aminopterin, 12
amniocentesis, 84
amoxicillin, 102–103
anencephaly, 5, 98
antibiotics
  allergies to, 194–195
  for ear infections, 199–201
  over use of, 190–192
  safety-net prescriptions, 200
anticonvulsant drugs, 89
antihistamines, 188, 195
Apgar, Virginia, Dr., 306–314
APGAR score, 306, 308–314
apnea, 60–61, 62, 69
apoptosis, 95–96
appendicitis
  mimicking conditions
    torsion or twisting of the right
      ovary, 218, 219
    tubal pregnancy, 261–262, 320
  peritonitis, 186, 187

signs and symptoms of, 187, 218
in toddlers, 186–187
arthritis, 3, 178
aspirin
fever and, 160, 167, 178, 188
Reye's syndrome, 167, 178
therapy, long-term, 189
asthma, 2, 189, 206
attention-behavioral problems, 26
Auckland, New Zealand, 52
autism, 243–244
Autism Society of America (ASA), 243–244

B
babies. *See* newborns and babies
The Baby Book (Sears and Sears), 182
"Baby in a Wicker Basket" (Stock), 343, 344
baby sitters, choosing, 151–152
baby's "lytes" (serum electrolytes), 173
Bactrim, 12
Ballard, Jean, 68
Baltimore Polytechnic Institute, 315
Beck, Joan, 312
Benfield, D. Gary, M. D., 314–316, 318–322
Bennett, Howard, M. D., 194
Bijani, Laleh and Landan, 293–294
bilirubin, 66
birth control pills. *See* contraceptives
birth defects
cousin couples, 87
critical periods of development, 27–29
defined, 100
detecting, before and after birth, 99–100
family history of, and genetics counseling, 9
herbal remedies, avoiding, 22
March of Dime's Birth Defects Section, 312
reference resources, 353
stigmas associated with, 313
see also neural tube defects (NTDs); *individual listings*
birth plans, 36, 41–43
blood pressure. *See* high blood pressure
Bogart, Humphrey, 65
Bogart, Maud, 65
Bogota, Colombia, 64
bones, and teen health, 271–273, 279
Botanical Safety Handbook (McGuffin), 8
bottle feeding
advantages, 152–153
baby bottle tooth decay, 161
intelligence *vs.* breastfeeding, 105–106
Bradley, Dr., 321–322
bradycardia, 60–61, 62
brain damage and disorders

brain death, defined, 304
cerebral palsy, 238–239
Ecstasy, recreational use of, 273–274
encephalitis, 198
Haemophilus influenzae type b, 177
herpes, genital, transmitted during delivery, 198
hydrocephalus, 5, 98
intraventricular hemorrhage (IVH), 61
oxygen deprivation, 48–49, 153, 216
Prozac and, 13–14, 114
respiratory function and, 60–61
shaken baby syndrome, 233–236
toxoplasmosis, 10
water births, 52–53
see also neural tube defects (NTDs)
brain development
breast milk's role in, 106
full maturity, and teen driving, 286–287
reading and, 148–149
right handedness, 61
speech control, 95
television, effects on, 184–185
Brazelton, T. Berry, M. D., 128
breastfeeding
bowel movements, in nursing babies, 111
breast implants, 103–104
breast reduction surgery, 104
cancer risks, lowering, 110
as contraceptive, 108–109
deciding on, influencing factors, 111–112, 143
father's support in, 112
flu, nursing with, 102
immunizations and, 102
intelligence, *vs.* bottle-feeding, 105–106
kangaroo-care mothers, 64
let-down reflex, 104
multiple sclerosis (MS), in nursing mother, 10
music, effects on, 109–110
pacifiers and, 123
planning for, 42, 62
in public, 105
reference resources, 348–349
second pregnancy, ease of *vs.* first pregnancy, 109
surgical procedures (biopsy, tumor/cyst removal), 104
see also breast milk
breast milk
amoxicillin, 102–103
caffeine, 21, 112–113
fatty acids, and brain development, 106
freezing for later use, 106–107
lithium-induced toxicity, 9, 103
phenobarbital, 110–111
propanalol, 105

Prozac, 13–14, 113–115
vitamin K, 119
of wet nurses, 107–108, 340
see also breastfeeding
breathing problems. *See* respiratory problems, in newborns
breech position, 46
Bresslau, Helene (Schweitzer), 317
bronchiolitis, 190
bronchitis, 191
bruises, 210–211
bubble blowing and drooling, 129–130
Budin, Pierre, Dr., 339–341
Bush, Barbara and Jenna, 80
Bush, George W., 80, 81, 298
Bush, Laura, 80, 81
Butterfield, Joseph, Dr., 312, 313–314

C

caffeine, 20–21, 112–113
calcium, 271–272, 279
cancer
 breast feeding, lowering the risk of, 110
 children with, talking to about death, 254–256
 drugs for, 8, 12
 lymphosarcoma, and intussusception, 215
 obesity, and risk of, 3
 penile, and circumcision, 73
 during pregnancy, treatments for, 294–296
 skin, and sun exposure, 240–242
candle burning, 230–231
carbamazepine, 8, 12
cataracts, 90
category X drugs, 14
cats, and pregnancy, 10–11
cells, 24, 84–85, 95–96
Center for Human Genetics (Boston University School of Medicine), 89
Centers for Disease Control (CDC), 3, 23, 180, 189
cerebral palsy (CP), 238–239
cesarean birth
 breastfeeding, 112
 doulas, 35
 elective, 30–32, 33, 34
 glucose levels of baby, 32–34
 rate of, 49–51, 69
 reasons for, 46–47, 54, 198
 respiratory problems in baby, 32–33, 34
 surgical procedure of
  risks, 31–32, 47
  step-by-step, 45–46
 vaginal birth after, 32, 50
Chang and Eng (Siamese twins), 81–82
Chicago's Century of Progress Exposition, 342

Chicago Tribune, 312
chickenpox (varicella)
 in adults, 198, 202
 "breakthrough" disease, 179
 complications from, 177–178, 198
 day care exclusion, AAP's criteria for, 233
 maternal, and fetal development (birth defects), 28, 29, 198
 pre-pregnancy checkup, testing for, 2
 scabbing and scars, 201–202
 see also immunizations
childbed fever (puerperal fever), 330–338
childbirth
 adjustment of babies at, 32–34
 birth plans, 36, 41–43
 education, 34–36, 306
 injuries during, 39–40
 problems, anticipating, 37–38, 47–49
 see also cesarean birth; labor and delivery
childproofing your home, 230
chlamydia infection, 197
choking, 153–154
 AAP recommended steps, 154
 "Top 10 Foods That Cause Choking," 173
chromosomes
 cell composition, 84
 Down syndrome, and extra chromosome #21, 84
 fragile X syndrome, 86–87
 gene for traits, 83
 hemophilia, and X chromosome, 116–117
 sex, 24, 86, 117
 in Turner syndrome patients, 281
circumcision
 AAP's policy on, 72–73
 benefits/disadvantages of, 73
 bleeding, and hemophilia, 115–117
 planning for, 42, 43, 74
 uncircumcised penis, care of, 74–75, 163–164
 warning bleeds, and vitamin K deficiency, 119
Clark, Mary Higgins, 87
cleft lip, 12, 89
cleft palate, 12, 89
Clinique Tarnier, 339–340
cloning, 96
coffee drinking, 20–21, 112–113
colds, common
 antibiotics for, 190–191
 calling the doctor, 188, 190
 decongestants, 188, 205, 266
 expectorants, 188
 and flu, differences in, 187–190
 prevalence of, 190, 192
 vaccine for, 90
 see also cough suppressants

colic, 70, 114, 140–142, 214
collar bone (clavicle) fractures, 39–40
Columbia Presbyterian Hospital, 307, 310, 312
Columbia University College of Physicians and Surgeons, 314
conceptual age, of fetus, 24–25
Coney Island, infant incubator exhibit, 339, 341, 342
congenital anomalies. *See* birth defects
conjunctivitis, and gonorrhea, 269
Contemporary Pediatrics, 119
contraceptives
  birth control pills, 8, 270
  breastfeeding as, 108–109
  St. John's wort, 8
  for teens, and parental consent, 263–264
Cord Blood Registry, 56
cough suppressants, 204–207
  dextromethorphan (DM), 205, 206
  diphenhydramine (DPH), 205, 206
  effectiveness of, research on, 205–206
  placebo effect, 206–207
Couney, Martin A., Dr. (Incubator-Baby Doctor), 338–343
cousin marriages, 87–88
Covey, M., Dr., 312
CPR, 154, 287–289
cradle cap (seborrhea), 209
crib safety, 222–224
Crick, Francis, 309
croup, 190, 206
Curtis, Glade B., M. D., 43
cyclopropane, 310
cystic fibrosis, 2, 84, 88, 292–293

D
decongestants, 188, 205, 266
DEET (N, N-diethyl-3–methylbenzamide), 203–204
delivery. *See* labor and delivery
depression
  drugs taken for, and pre-pregnancy concerns, 2, 8
  father factor in child development, 134
  lithium, 8–9
  obesity and, 3, 275
  see also Prozac
Desmond, Murdina, M. D., 309–310
developmental biology, 96
diabetes
  cesarean birth, necessity for, 46
  in children
    complications of, 276–277
    obesity and, 275, 276–278
    sports participation and, 260–261
    symptoms of, 278
  in Down syndrome patients, 90
  explained, 276

flu shots, 189
hyperglycemia, 276–277
inheritability of, 1
pre-pregnancy concerns, 5–7
  controlling, 2
  counseling, preconceptual, 5–8
  obesity, 3
stem cell research, 297
  in Turner's syndrome patients, 282
types of, 277
Diamond-Blackfan anemia, 290
diaper pails, precautions, 163
diaper rash, 207–208
diaphragmatic hernia, 99
diarrhea, 166, 196, 232, 280
dihydrofolate reductase inhibitors, 12
Dilantin
  cleft lip and cleft palate, incidence of, 89
  fetal development, effect on, 28
  folic acid, effect on, 12
  pre-pregnancy concerns, 2
  St. John's wort, drug interaction, 8
DNA
  double helix structure, 309
  fragile X syndrome, 86
  genetic disorders, 1–2
  learning about, through developmental biology, 96
Dole, Robert, 329
doulas, 34–36
Doulas of North America, 36
Down syndrome
  cause of, and chromosome #21, 84
  health problems associated with, 89–90, 93
  life expectancy, 72, 89–90
  long-term care, after death of caregiver(s), 89, 299–300
  risk of having a baby with, 85
  signs of, 93
Dr. Spock's Baby and Child Care (Spock), 147, 182, 322, 325
drooling and bubble blowing, 129–130
drowning
  in bath water, 160, 162, 221
  in diaper pails, 163
  rates of, in U. S., 222
  swimming lessons, 221–222

E
E. coli infection, 232
ear infections
  antibiotic treatments, 199–201
  bottle feeding in bed, 161
  composition of ear, 193
  examining for, 194
  hearing loss from, 194
  otitis externa, 193

otitis media (middle ear infection), 194, 199, 200, 201
swimmer's ear, 193, 194
Ecstasy, 273–274
electrical shock, and fetal death, 15
embryology, 96
embryo tissue-typing, 290, 291
emergency childbirth, 38–39
encephalitis, 178, 198
"An Enemy of the People" (Ibsen), 338
epilepsy. *See* seizure disorders
epinephrine, 195
expectorants, 188
eye infections and disorders
   blocked tear ducts, 162
   chlamydia and, 197
   conjunctivitis, and gonorrhea, 269
   glaucoma, 90
   purulent conjunctivitis, 233–234

F
Factor VIII, 116–117
Factor IX, 116–117
falls, on stairs, 236–237
Fanconi's Anemia, 57
Farrow, Mathew, 57
fertilization, 24
fetal development
   breathing, in the womb, 26–27
   cells, and amniocentesis, 84
   critical periods of, 27–29
   gestational age *vs.* conceptual age, 24–25
   intrauterine growth retardation, 25–26
   monitoring, 16–18, 42
   radiation exposure, 27, 28
   sex of baby, determining, 24
   stunted growth, and cigarette smoking, 19–20
fever, 159–160
   alcohol sponge baths for, 159
   aspirin for, 160, 167, 178, 188
   temperature, taking, 166
First Congregational Church of Akron, 244
flu. *See* influenza (flu)
fluorescent light (phototherapy), 65–67
folate
   and folic acid, differences between, 96–97
   sources of, 5
   and vitamin B, 96, 98
folic acid
   inhibiting drugs, and birth defects, 11–13
   multivitamins for, 2, 5, 7, 11, 13, 97, 98–99
   see also folate; neural tube defects (NTDs)

Food and Drug Administration (FDA), 8, 114
fragile X syndrome, 85–87
Friedman, Pauline Esther and Esther Pauline (Ann Landers and "Dear Abby"), 80–81

G
gays and lesbians, as parents, 171–172
gene mutations
   apoptosis, 95–96
   for cystic fibrosis, 84
   for fragile X syndrome, 86
   inherited diseases, 2
   for situs inversus, 95
   for syndactyly, 95
genetic disorders
   cousin couples and risk of, 87
   newborn autopsy, for detecting, 247
   pre-pregnancy check-up, for detecting, 1–2
   reference resources, 353
   revealing to relatives, moral obligations, 292–293
   in teen, dealing with, 280–282
   see also inherited diseases
genetics
   counselor, 9, 87, 88, 117, 249
   dominant-recessive genes, 83
   genone, 84–85
   reference resources, 353
   science of, 96
   see also DNA
genitals, 181–183
German measles (rubella)
   maternal, and fetal development, 28
   pre-pregnancy checkup, testing for, 2
   vaccine, and childhood immunizations, 176
gestational age
   conceptual age and, 24–25
   corrected, 61
   determining, methods of, 67–68
      after birth assessment, 68
      judgment errors in, 67–68
      ultrasound, 17–18, 68
   large for gestational age (LGA), 68, 173
   small for gestational age, 68
Gilbert, Ruth, Dr., 53
glaucoma, 90
glucose levels, 32–34, 260, 276–278
gonorrhea, 267–269

D. Gary Benfield, M.D.

grandparents
   first time grandmother, 170
   support given by, 174–176
   understanding new grandchild, 168–170
Grant, Cary (Leach, Archibald), 342–343

H

H. flu. *See* Haemophilus influenzae type b
Hack, Maureen, Dr., 90
Haemophilus influenzae type b, 177
Hale, Thomas, Ph. D., 115
Harper, Barbara, 52, 53
head lice, 233, 256–259
   AAP's recommendations
      for day care exclusion, 232, 256–257, 259
      "no nit policy" (Web site link), 258
      for treatment, 257, 259
   in African Americans, 259
   diagnosing, 259
   effect of, on scalp, 258–259
   forms of, 258
   transmission of, 259
hearing loss, 90, 194, 282
heart defects
   critical periods of development, 28, 29
   dihydrofolate reductase inhibitors, 12
   electrical shock, and fetal cardiac arrest, 15
   lithium-induced toxicity, 103
   situs Inversus, 94–95
   in Turner syndrome patients, 282
heart disease
   cesarean births, and necessity for, 46
   congenital, 93, 164, 245, 267
   drugs for, and St. John's wort, 8
   flu shot recommendations, 189
   Haemophilus influenzae type b, infections caused by, 177
   heart attack
      and Ecstasy use, 274
      and NEC, 216
   hyperglycemia, 276
   murmurs, 93, 164–165
   obesity, and risk of, 3, 275, 276, 279
heart rate
   in adults, 70
   anesthesia, effect on, 309
   APGAR score, 312
   bradycardia, 60–61, 62
   Ecstasy use, 273
   fetal, 17, 20
   heat stroke, 284
   lithium-induced toxicity, 103
   in newborns, 48, 70, 71
   in toddlers, 186
heat related illnesses
   children left in cars, 160, 285
   heat cramps, 283
   heat exhaustion, 283–284
   heat stroke, 160, 284–285
   salt depletion, 283
   tips for athletes, 285
hemangiomas, 211–212
   strawberry, 212
hemophilia, 115–117
hepatitis, 177, 178, 233
herbs
   avoiding during pregnancy, 7, 22
   fenugreek, 7–8
   pennyroyal, 21–22
   St. John's wort, 8
heredity. *See* inherited diseases
herpes, genital, 46, 197–198
Hess, Julius, Dr., 340
high blood pressure
   cesarean birth, necessity for, 46
   in children, 266–267, 275
   inheritability of, 1
   obesity, 275, 279
   pre-pregnancy checkup, 1, 2
   pseudoephedrine, effect on, 266–267
   types of, 267
   "white coat" effect, 266
HIV infection, 22–23, 28, 73
Hutchins, Carleen, 311–312
hyaline membrane disease, 58
hydrocephalus, 5, 98
hyperactivity, 26
hyperbaric oxygen, 238–239
hyperglycemia, 276–277
hypertension. *See* high blood pressure
hypothermia, 69
hypothyroidism, 16

I

Ibsen, Henrik, 338
ibuprofen, 160, 188
IDM (infant of a diabetic mother), 173
immune globulin, 179
immunizations
   breastfeeding and, 102
   for chickenpox (varicella), 177–178, 198
   complications from, 179, 202
   and pregnancy, 179
   for colds, 176
   for German measles (rubella), 176
   necessity of, 176–177
   for smallpox, 179–180
impetigo, 212–213, 233
Incubator-Baby Doctor (Couney, Martin A., Dr.), 338–343

infertility
  caffeine, heavy consumption of, 112
  cesarean birth, 32
  fertility clinics, and frozen embryos, 297
  gonorrhea, 269
  PID, 268, 269
influenza (flu)
  and colds, differences in, 187–190
  flu season, 190
  shot recommendations for, 189, 190
  symptoms of, 189
inherited diseases
  cystic fibrosis, 2, 84, 88, 292–293
  diabetes, 1
  hemophilia, 116
  high blood pressure, 1
  learning about, through developmental biology, 96
  mental retardation, 86
  muscular dystrophy, 116
  seizure disorders, 1
  sickle sell anemia, 2, 90–91
insect bites, 203–204
Institute of Health (London), 53
intelligence
  breastfeeding, *vs.* bottle-feeding, 105–106
  of children with lesbian, gay parents, 171
  CP, 239
  father factor in development and, 147
  of firstborn children, 108–109
  IQ quiz, for newborn, 69–71
  premature infants, 90
  smoking during pregnancy, 20
  of Turner syndrome patients, 282
intestine
  diaphragmatic hernia, 99
  folic acid absorption, 97
  intussusception, 214
  NEC, 215–217
  perforations of small, and falls, 236–237
  phenobarbital absorption, 110
intrauterine growth retardation, 25–26
intussusception, 214–215
in vitro fertilization, 80, 282, 290–291
Isaac Asimov's Book of Facts, 132
Is My Baby Alright?: A 1973 Guide to Birth Defects (Apgar and Beck), 312–313

J
jaundice, and phototherapy, 65–67
Jefferson Davis Hospital (Houston), 309
John Hopkins University, 312
Journal of Pediatrics, 195
Journal of the American Medical Association (JAMA), 90, 290, 312, 343

K
kangaroo care, 64–65
Kant's Philosophy of Religion (Schweitzer), 317
Kennedy, Arabella, 59
Kennedy, Caroline, 59
Kennedy, Jacqueline, 57–59
Kennedy, John, F., Jr., 57–58
Kennedy, John F., 59
Kennedy, Patrick, 57–58
kidneys
  chickenpox vaccine complications, 178
  diabetes and, 276
  Potter's syndrome, 248, 249
King, Martin Luther, 322
Klein, Professor, 333, 335
Kolletschka, Dr., 332–333
Krantz, John, Dr., 206

L
labor and delivery
  boys, and length of labor, 37
  contractions, and lung fluid, 33
  forceps usage, 31, 35, 41, 186
  large babies, delivery of, 47
  onset of, guidelines for, 38–39
  premature, 18, 20, 58, 78
  prolonged, 46
  suction cup usage, 40–41
  water breaking, 38, 47
  see also childbirth
Lambarene, 317, 318
Lancet, 109
laser treatments, for tattoo removal while pregnant, 18–19
Leach, Archibald (Grant, Cary), 342–343
left-handedness, 126
let-down reflex, 104
leukemia, 89, 289, 290, 292
LGA (large for gestational age), 173
lithium, 8–9, 103
liver
  Ecstasy, and failure of, 274
  glucose production by, 34
  Reyes syndrome, failure of, 167, 178
  situs inversus, 95
loss of a child
  advice given by others, 250
  conceiving again, afterwards, 248–249
  dying child, talking about death with, 254–257
  newborn autopsy, 246–248
  physician's mishandling of, and bereavement, 251–253
  reference resources, 353–355
  remembering deceased children, 244–246
  siblings and, 250–251

lupus, 11
Lupus Foundation of America, 11

M
M. D. Anderson Cancer Center (Houston), 296
March of Dimes
 APGAR score, and Virginia Apgar, 312–314
 Bereavement Kit, 354
 Birth Defects Section of, 312
 genetics counseling, 9
 resource materials from, 345, 353, 354
Martin, Cindy, 306, 314
masturbation, 183
May, Annabelle (Couney), 341
McInnerney, Connor Shamus, 300–304
measles, 233
 see also German measles (rubella)
medical history, and pre-pregnancy checkup, 1–2
Medical Quality Assurance Commission (Washington), 302
Medical University of Budapest, 338
Medications and Mothers' Milk (Hale), 115
meningitis, 177, 178
mental retardation
 chickenpox, maternal, 29
 CP, 239
 family support, 94
 fragile X syndrome, 86
 heat exhaustion, 283
 intrauterine growth retardation, 25–26
 masturbation, myth of, 183
methotrexate, 12
Michael Reese Hospital (Chicago), 340
Mills, Victor, 208
Milunsky, Aubrey, M. D., 89
miscarriage
 caffeine, heavy consumption of, 112
 diabetes, 6
 herbal remedies to avoid, 21–22
 hypothyroidism, 16
 Prozac, 13
 smoking, 20
Missing Children's Assistance Act, 224–225
Mitchtom, Morris, 44
mongolian spots, 209–210, 211
multiple births
 cesarean births, 47
 problems at delivery, anticipating, 37–38
 reference resources, 352
 separate deliveries of, 77–78
 triplets, 47, 80
 in vitro fertilization, 80
 see also twins
multiple pregnancies, and pre-pregnancy checkup, 2

multiple sclerosis, 9–10
mumps, 233
muscular dystrophy, 2
The Mystery of the Kingdom of God (Schweitzer), 317

N
National Association of School Nurses, 259
National Candle Association, 231
National Center for Missing and Exploited Children, 228
National Fire Protection Association (NFPA), 230, 231
National Gallery of Art, 344
necrotizing enterocolitis (NEC), 215–217
neural tube defects (NTDs)
 anencephaly, 5, 98
 encephalocele, 98
 folic acid, and multivitamins, 2, 5, 7, 11, 13, 97, 98–99
 neural tube development, explained, 4–5, 97–98
 spina bifida, 2, 4–5, 98
newborns and babies
 adjustment of, at childbirth, 32–34
 air travel, 120–121
 baby food, 134–135
  microwave heating of, 221
 baby sitters, choosing, 151–152
 bathing
  frequency of, 162
  leaving unattended, 160, 162, 221
  urinating in water, 145–147
 birth weight
  influencing factors, 19–20, 112
  slow weight gain, 20, 114
  of term babies *vs* premature, 68
 books, introducing to, 130–131, 148–149
 childproofing your home, 230
 crawling, dangers of, 228–230
 crying, 128–129, 154–157
 drooling and bubble blowing, 129–130
 eye sight of, 215
 love for baby, beginning feelings of, 142–144
 reference resources, 349–352
 room temperature for, 165
 siblings, and adjustment to, 144–145
 sleep
  average hours per day, 72
  bedding precautions, 125
  crib safety, 222–224
  positions, 124–125
  REM and non-REM, 136–139, 169–170
  "sleeping through the night," defined, 138–139
  states of, 169–170
  twitching and jerking during, 139

soft spot, 165–166
solid foods, introducing, 134–135
   microwave heating of, 221
states of consciousness, 169–170
statistical information, 71–72
stranger anxiety, 131
teeth
   baby bottle tooth decay, 161
   brushing, 167–168
   dental visits, 168
   first, 127
temperament, 139–140
vaginal bleeding in, 117
vitamin supplements, need for, 163
walking
   before crawling, 128
   first steps, and age, 125–126
   limping, after falling, 40
   shoes and, 130
   walkers, dangers of, 220–221
see also parents; respiratory problems, in newborns
New England Journal of Medicine, 12, 13, 203
The New York Times, 296, 338
Ngai, S. H., M. D., 310
NIX (permethrin), 257, 259
Nuland, Sherwin B., M. D., 337

O
obesity
   birth defect risks, 3
   in children
      conditions associated with, 275
      gastric bypass for teenagers, 278–280
      psychological stress of, 276
   health risks, 3
   heredity, 275
   teen health and, 274–276
   see also diabetes
Ocean City, Maryland, 263
Olympic Memorial Hospital (Port Angeles), 300, 302
omphalocele, 3
open spine defects. *See* spina bifida
The Orange County Register, 327
Out of My Life and Thought (Schweitzer), 316, 318
ovary, torsion or twisting of, 217–219

P
pacifiers, 123
Papper, E. M., Dr., 308
parents
   allergy histories of, 194–195
   attention given by, 149–150
   father factor in child development, 132–134, 147
   lesbian and gay, 171
   preference for one parent over the other, 129, 150
   single, U. S. Census Bureau statistics, 172
   stay-at-home, 157–159
   STDs, and consent for treatment, 264
Paris Maternity Hospital, 339–340
Paris Missionary Society, 317
Paxil, 2, 115
Peale, Norman Vincent, 322
pediatricians
   choosing, 152
   fees, 43–44
   terminology used by, 173
pelvic inflammatory disease (PID), 268–269
penicillin, 194, 195, 196
Pennsylvania State College of Medicine, 205–206
pennyroyal, 21–22
peritonitis, 186, 187, 216, 217
permethrin (NIX), 257, 259
phenobarbital
   breastfeeding precautions, 110–111
   folic acid, effect on, 12
   pre-pregnancy concerns, 2
   St. John's wort, drug interaction, 8
Philosophy of Civilization (Schweitzer), 317
photodermatitis, 211
phototherapy, 65–67
Physician's Desk Reference (PDR), 113–114
Picasso, Pablo, 132
pneumonia, 177, 190, 197, 198, 206
poison ivy, 213–214
Potter, Edith, Dr., 248, 249
Potter's syndrome, 248–249
pregnancy
   counseling, 89
   full-term baby, defined, 67–68
   love for baby, beginning feelings of, 142–144
   overdue, 54
   planning, reference resources, 345
   teens and, 269–271
   unwed mothers, U. S. statistics on, 126–127
preimplantation genetic diagnosis, 290, 291
premature birth
   APGAR score, and Virginia Apgar, 312–314
   apnea, 60–61
   baby care, 59–61
   bradycardia, 60–61
   challenges of, 61–63
   diabetes, 6
   discharge from hospital, 62–63
   gestational age assessment, 67–69

Incubator-Baby Doctor, 338–343
intraventricular hemorrhage (IVH), 60, 61
jaundice, and fluorescent light treatment, 65–67
kangaroo care, 64–65
lupus, 11
massage therapy, 63
NEC, 216–217
neurological damage, long-term follow-up studies, 90
obesity, 3
percent of in U.S.A., according to race, 72
prevention, medical advances in, 58
reference resources, 346–348, 349
respiratory distress syndrome (RDS), 60
smoking, 11
sudden infant death syndrome (SIDS), 235–236
vitamin requirements, 163
pre-pregnancy checkup, 1–3
primidone, 12
Proctor & Gamble, 208
propanalol, 105
Prozac
   breastfeeding while taking, 14, 113–115
   maternal benefits *vs.* fetal risks, 13–14
   pre-pregnancy concerns, 2
pseudoephedrine, 266
puerperal fever (childbed fever), 330–338
purulent conjunctivitis, 233–234
Pushnik, Frieda, 326–327
pyrimethamine, 12

Q
The Quest of the Historical Jesus (Schweitzer), 317

R
rapid eye movement (REM), 136–139, 169–170
reading
   books, introducing to newborns and babies, 130–131, 148–149
   brain development, 148–149
   crisis, AAP on, 148
   on a daily basis, 181
   to older children, 150–151
Red Cross
   Bone Marrow Donor Program, 290
   CPR classes, 154
Reproductive Genetics Institute, 290

reptiles, as pets
   iguanas, 195–196
   rules for owning, 196
   salmonella bacteria, 195–196
   turtles, 196–197
resource center
   baby and child care, 349–352
   breastfeeding, 348–349
   genetics and birth defects, 353
   perinatal loss, 353–355
   planning your pregnancy, 345
   pregnancy, 345–346
   premature birth, 346–348
   twins and higher multiples, 352
respiratory distress syndrome (RDS), 60
respiratory problems, in newborns
   APGAR score, 312
   apnea, 60–61, 62, 69
   cesarean births, and babies, 32–33, 34
   choking, 153–154
   diabetic mothers, 44
   diaphragmatic hernia, 99
   hyaline membrane disease, 58
   oxygen deprivation, at birth, 48–49
   RDS, 60
   resuscitation, in delivery room, 37–38, 43, 49
   unilateral choanal artresia, 100–102
   upper respiratory infections, 191–192, 205, 266
   see also sudden infant death syndrome (SIDS)
resuscitation
   in delivery room, 37–38, 43, 49
   ethical questions, 300–304
Reye's syndrome, 167, 178
rhinitis, allergic, 206
ringworm, 212–213
Ripley, Robert, 326, 327
Roach, Laurel, 281–282
Rochford General Hospital, 66
Roosevelt, Eleanor, 328
Roosevelt, Franklin Delano, 328–329
Royal Children's Hospital (Bristol, England), 109
rubella. *See* German measles (rubella)

S
Saint Roche's Hospital, 336
St. John's wort, 8
Sallie and Adelaide (wives of Chang and Eng), 82
salmonella infection, 195–196
scabies, 233
Schweitzer, Albert, Dr., 314, 316–322
Sears, William and Martha, 182
seborrhea (cradle cap), 209

seizure disorders
  epilepsy, 12, 110, 183
  inheritability of, 1
  inhibiting drugs, and birth defects, 11–13
  masturbation, myths and, 183
  see also Dilantin
Semmelweis, Ignaz, Dr., 329–338
sex
  of baby, determining, 24
  during pregnancy, 18
sexually transmitted diseases (STDs)
  abstinence, 270
  circumcision, 73
  gonorrhea, 268–269
  herpes, genital, 46, 197–198
  parental consent for treatment, 264
shaken baby syndrome
  brain damage caused by, 233–236
  as child abuse, proving, 234–236
  described, 234
Shigella infection, 232
short bowel syndrome (short gut), 217
sickle cell disease, 2, 90–91
SIDS. *See* sudden infant death syndrome (SIDS)
sinus infection, 186, 206
situs inversus, 95
smallpox, 179–180
"Smart Guide to Kid's TV" (AAP Web site), 185
Smith, Dr., 321–322
smoking
  adverse effects of, 2, 20
  low birth weight, 19, 20, 113
  nicotine replacement therapy, 20
  smoke ingredients, 19
sore throat, 186, 189, 190
  strep throat, 233
spanking, 147
Sparky the Fire Dog, 230–231
sperm, 24
spina bifida, 2, 4–5, 98, 314
Spock, Benjamin, M. D., 147, 182, 322–326
Spock, Mildred, 322, 323
Springer, Korey, 284
stem cell research
  "Alaya method," 290
  controversy over, 291–292, 297–298
  embryo tissue-typing, 290, 291
  government funding for, 297–298
  preimplantation genetic diagnosis, 290, 291
  umbilical cord blood, 54–57, 290, 298
  in vitro fertilization, 290–291
stillbirth
  diabetes, 6
  hypothyroidism, 16
  obesity, 3

Prozac, 13
support groups, 354
Stock, Joseph, 343–344
stranger anxiety, 131
strep throat, 233
Striegel-Wilson, Jana, 296
sudden infant death syndrome (SIDS)
  AAP
    "Back to Sleep" campaign, 122
    prevention guidelines, 121–123, 125
  cause of, 122
  side sleeping, 124–125
  smoking during pregnancy, 20
  statistics, 122
  tummy time, 123, 124
sulfasalazine, 12
sunburn
  African Americans and, 242–243
  preventing, 240, 241–242, 243
  signs of, 242
  skin cancer, 241
  sunscreen, and SPF ratio, 240, 242
  treatment for, 242
  ultraviolet rays, and foggy/hazy days, 241
sunscreen, and SPF ratio, 240, 242
Swain, Joseph, Dr., 343, 344
syndactyly, 95
Synthroid, 16

T

tattoos, removing while pregnant, 18–19
tear ducts, blocked, 161–162
teen health
  alcohol consumption, 228, 262–263, 287
  blood pressure, 266–267
  bones, 271–273
  driving, 285–287
  Ecstasy use, 273–274
  emancipated minor, defined, 264–265
  gonorrhea, 267–269
  inclusion in health discussions, 264
  obesity, 274–276
  pregnancy, discussing with, 269–271
  prescription contraceptives, and parental consent, 263–264
  tattoos and body piercings, and parental consent, 265–266
  television viewing, of children under age 2, 183–185
    brain development, effects on, 184–185
    "Smart Guide to Kid's TV" (AAP), 185
thyroid disorders
  in Down syndrome patients, 90
  hypothyroidism, and Synthroid, 16
  thyroiditis, and Turner syndrome patients, 282

toddlers
  bad breath of, 185–186
  genitals, discovery of, 181–183
  heart rate of, 186
  negative behavior, 180–181
  nose, inserting objects up, 185–186
  self-comforting habits, 183
  spanking, 147
  swallowing coins, 219–220
  television and, 183–185
  toe-sucking, 127–128
  vocabulary, 124
  see also newborns and babies
toe-sucking, 127–128
tongue-thrust reflex, 134–135
tonsillitis, 186
Topel, Amy, 278–279
toxoplasmosis, 10
TPN (total parenteral nutrition), 173
traits, genes and, 83
triamterene, 12
trimethoprim, 12
tubal pregnancy, 261–262, 320
tuberculosis, 233
tummy time, 123, 124
Turner, Eugene, 301–304
twins
  celebrity, 80–82
  conjoined, 79, 80, 293–294
  fraternal, 78–80
  identical
    mood disorders, and genes, 75–76
    raising, 76–77
  incident rates of, 72
  Siamese, 79, 80, 81–82, 327
  vanishing twin syndrome, 75
  see also multiple births
Tylenol Sinus, 266

U
U. S. Centers for Disease Control and Prevention (CDC), 3, 23, 180, 189
ultrasound, fetal
  fetal number, deterring, 18
  gestational age, deterring, 17–18
  heart pulsations, visibility of, 17
  neural tube defects (NTDs), diagnosis of, 5
  procedure, method of, 17
  sound, principles of, 16–17
umbilical cord
  cesarean birth and, 46, 47
  emergency childbirth procedures and, 39

fetal circulation and, 55
omphalocele, 3
stem cell research and, 54–57, 290, 298
unilateral choanal artresia, 100–102
University of Cincinnati, 200
University of Maryland School of Medicine (Baltimore), 321–322
upper respiratory infections, 191–192, 205, 266
  see also colds, common
urinary tract defects, 12
urinary tract infections (UTIs), 73, 217, 218

V
vaginal bleeding, in newborn, 117
Vienna General Hospital, 330, 331, 335, 336
Virchow, Rudolph, 337
vitamins
  B, 96, 98
  D, 163, 271–273
  for folic acid, 2, 5, 7, 11, 13, 97, 98–99
  K deficiency, 119
  for newborns and babies, need for, 163

W
walking
  before crawling, 128
  first steps, and age, 125–126
  limping, after falling, 40
  shoes and, 130
  walkers, dangers of, 220–221
Washington Medical Center, 319, 321
water birth, 52–53
Watson, James, 309
Whipple, Allen, Dr., 307
White, Franklin, 343
whooping cough, 233
"withdrawal" bleeding, 117

Y
Yale University, 323
  rowing team, 323–325
"You and Your Family" (AAP Web site), 185
Your Pregnancy: Questions and Answers (Curtis), 43

Z
zidovudine (Retrovir), 23
Zoloft, 115